WHOLE
BEAUTY

SHIVA ROSE

WHOLE BEAUTY

Daily Rituals and Natural Recipes for Lifelong Beauty and Wellness

Photographs by
NGOC MINH NGO

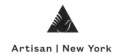

Artisan | New York

Library of Congress Cataloging-in-Publication Data
Names: Rose, Shiva, author
Title: Whole beauty : Daily rituals and natural recipes for lifelong beauty and wellness / Shiva Rose
Description: New York : Artisan, a division of Workman Publishing Co., Inc. [2018] | Includes an index.
Identifiers: LCCN 2017037796 | ISBN 9781579657727 (hc : alk. paper) | ISBN 9781579658700 (special edition)
Subjects: LCSH: Beauty, Personal. | Women—Health and hygiene. | Self-care, Health
Classification: LCC RA778 .R6185 2018 | DDC 646.7/2—dc23
LC record available at https://lccn.loc.gov/2017037796

Cover design by Michelle Ishay-Cohen
Cover photographs by Ngoc Minh Ngo
Cover illustrations by Spiros Halaris
Book design by CHD

Artisan books are available at special discounts when purchased in bulk for premiums and
sales promotions as well as for fund-raising or educational use. Special editions or book
excerpts also can be created to specification. For details, contact the Special Sales Director
at the address below, or send an e-mail to specialmarkets@workman.com.

For speaking engagements, contact speakersbureau@workman.com.

Published by Artisan
A division of Workman Publishing Co., Inc.
225 Varick Street
New York, NY 10014-4381
artisanbooks.com

Artisan is a registered trademark of Workman Publishing Co., Inc.

Published simultaneously in Canada by Thomas Allen & Son, Limited

Printed in China

3 5 7 9 10 8 6 4 2

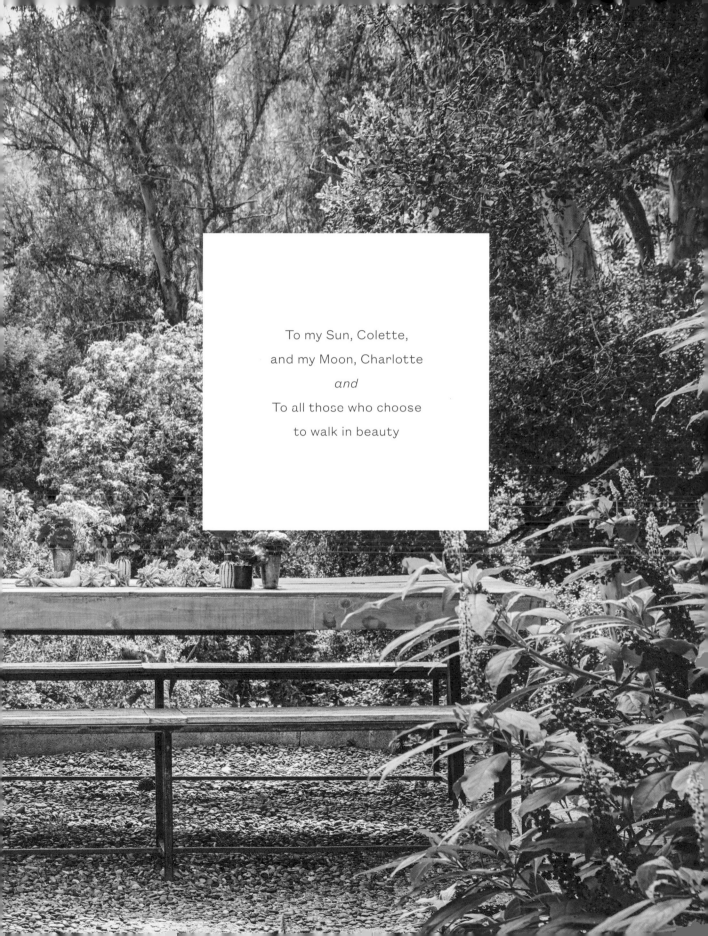

To my Sun, Colette,
and my Moon, Charlotte
and
To all those who choose
to walk in beauty

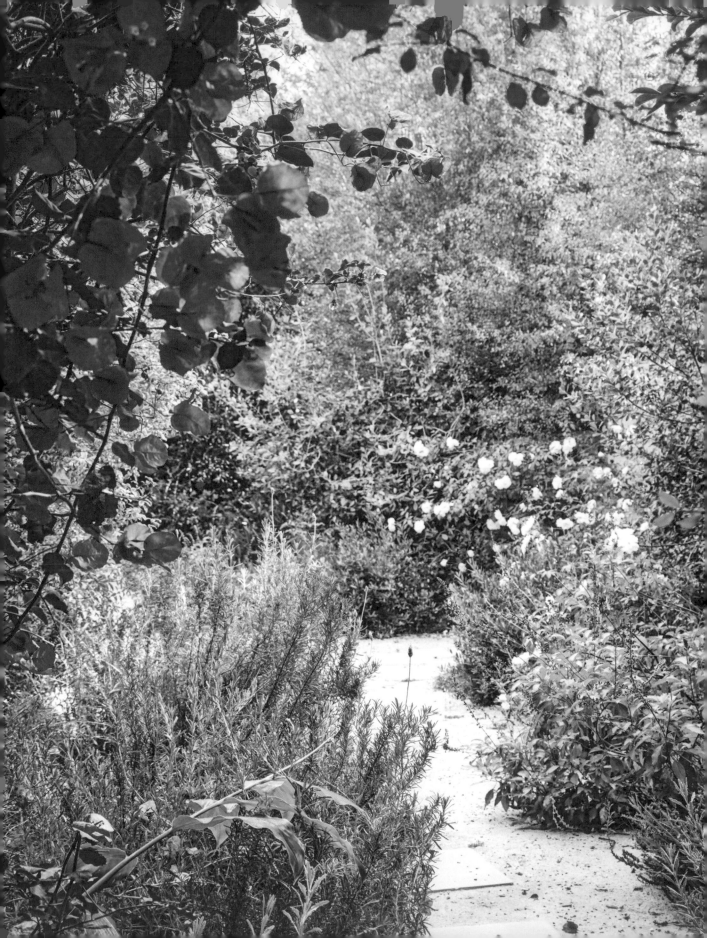

CONTENTS

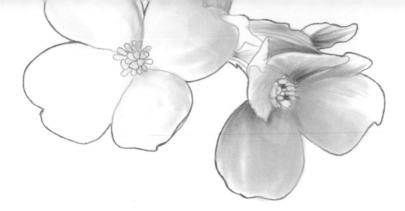

PREFACE

I spend hours in our garden, gathering pansies, roses, cherry blossoms, and all the other vivid, scented plants that catch my eye. I collect the petals in a small copper bowl, add a little water from the pond, and with a pestle, mash them until they form a fragrant and vibrant paste.

I take my seat at the edge of the pond and dangle my feet in, piquing the curiosity of the goldfish, sending them swimming to ripple the lily pads across the surface.

I take my flower paste and rub it on my face, breathing in the aroma of the flowers. This is Iran, this is the beginning, but if I close my eyes now, many years and thousands of miles away in Los Angeles, I am there again. I can still feel the wind on my cheeks and the tickle of fish nibbling at my toes and hear birds singing as they dance by overhead.

I was young enough that I didn't think of these pondside rituals as beautifying or acts of self-care. I just saw them as a way to bring myself even closer to the natural world, reveling in the way the yellows, reds, and purples looked before my eyes and how soft the petals felt as I crushed them with my hands. It was a pure moment of creation that amplified my senses and gave me a small gift of beauty to carry with me even when I was called away from the garden to tend to my chores or go to bed.

The first several decades of my life were marked by trauma. In 1979, due to the Iranian Revolution, my family was in danger, my mother being an American citizen and my father a well-known liberal TV personality. They felt it was best that we leave the country, so we escaped Tehran on one of the last flights out. We resettled in Los Angeles, where my parents had a lot of tumultuous times before they divorced when I was a teenager. Not long after that, one of my closest friends was murdered on her way home from a party we attended together. To escape these challenging times, I immersed myself in acting, eventually going on to study theater at UCLA.

I married young and gave birth to my first daughter, Colette Blu, in my midtwenties. Motherhood hit me hard in ways I did not expect. I was achy and tired all the time, and the dark circles under my eyes were visible from a mile away. I was juggling being a mom, being a wife to a successful actor, and pursuing a career as an actress. I kept waiting for a bounce-back that never came. I eventually went to a doctor, not because of how I was feeling but because of a bruise that appeared on my back. That was when I was diagnosed with scleroderma, lupus, and rheumatoid arthritis and told

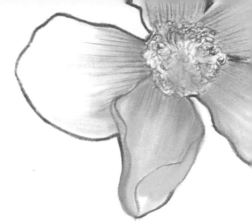

that unless I took drastic measures, I might not have more than a year to live.

This was a fate I refused to accept, and I began the process of healing myself through organic foods, herbal medicines, Ayurveda, self-care, and adding healthy fats to my diet. Though my quality of life was less than optimal, I improved. I learned how to manage my symptoms and live with chronic pain. I didn't realize how much pain I was in until years and years later when it subsided. At the time, I counted this minor relief as a small success.

Then in 2008, the perfect storm hit and blew everything to pieces. I had just given birth to my second daughter, Charlotte Rumi Rose; my sixteen-year marriage was crumbling; and to top it off, I was being sued for trying to save a two-hundred-year-old oak tree. Due to all of this stress, my symptoms began to return.

One night, I finally broke. Wearing nothing but a slip, I ran barefoot out of my house into the darkness, not sure that I could handle my life anymore. I was running from my marriage, running from the fractured life that I had created, running from my illness, running from childhood traumas, just running.

I'd been running for an hour when the thought of my baby daughter stopped me. Her face, her violet-blue eyes, propelled me to turn back. This time was undoubtedly

my darkest moment, but in that abyss, something bright still glimmered. My maternal instincts compelled me, but I also drew strength from the courageous women of my family's past—the mothers, wives, and daughters of nomads who had crossed the mountains of Persia—and from the powerful combination of my Euro/American lineage: the Native American blood on my mother's side along with that of the hardy souls of my English ancestors. I knew that they were watching me and urging me on. They had known trauma; they had known grief. They had survived, and so would I.

The only good thing about hitting rock bottom is that you have nowhere to go but up, and as I limped home that night—declining a ride from a kind neighbor who saw me and pulled over to the side of the road—I knew it was time to wipe the slate clean. I could choose to treat my anxiety and depression, which were symptoms of my pain, or I could face the pain and overhaul my being. I chose to do the latter, because I knew that I didn't just want to survive, I wanted to thrive.

I had to start over from an earthier place, burn the house down and rebuild. I got divorced, and I didn't take much with me—clothes, books, a poster. I set about finding a new house for my tiny tribe: my daughters and myself. I didn't know where we would land, but I knew that we had to be surrounded by green.

In Iran, I had grown up near the mountains. Close by were bustling markets—a far cry from the supermarkets of America—and bursting gardens, and I resolved to reestablish that connection to the natural world. I wanted to dig my fingers into the earth. I found solace in feeling and smelling the soil. I grew my own vegetables and learned how to compost. I then began raising chickens and eventually honeybees.

Everything that followed was a natural progression. I focused on being in rhythm with the cycles and seasons of nature. I started to make my own skin-care and cleaning products. Inspired by my new philosophy, I was drawn to a community of like-minded people who had a similar ethos. Overhauling my life and sharing my experiences became my work, and I realized that I was doing what I loved. Once you are on your true path, opportunities will present themselves; the important thing is being open enough to recognize them.

I started my blog, *The Local Rose*, because I wanted to share and document what I was doing. I met all of these incredible practitioners along the way as I was changing my life, and discovered that there were a lot of us searching for inspiration. I wanted to show that it was possible to be green and conscious and still be chic, and have a platform to talk about what was important to me without being preachy. At the time, almost eight years ago, natural beauty was mostly relegated to health food stores, and was seen as mundane cleansing rather than pampering. I felt like it deserved to have the same elevated elegance of the luxurious (yet often highly toxic) products from high-end beauty counters. As women began to come to me with questions or to share their own stories, I realized that while my journey was a personal endeavor, the benefits of it radiated far beyond me.

In our modern, fast-paced era, women are stressed and under more pressure than ever before, and as a result have lost the essence of being sensual in many ways. Sensuality is about having a connection to yourself, your soul, the luscious fruit that goes into your face mask, the music that makes you want to dance, the wind caressing your cheek—indulging in all the things that make you feel alive and beautiful. Approaching beauty with reverence and ritual can help awaken your feminine fire and stoke the flames of vibrancy and passion. Beauty and self-care nourish us so that we can continue to give to others.

I truly believe that beautifying ourselves holistically is an integral part of self-care, health, and healing. When we treat our body, our vessel, with intention, we are honoring not just ourselves but the essence of femininity that has coursed through us since the beginning of time.

I hope to inspire you to start on your own wellness journey and to not give up as you traverse the peaks and valleys. The process is not linear. In art and architecture, there is a belief that things that have straight lines with defined beginnings and endings are masculine, whereas the feminine is represented by spirals, curves, and circular forms. This is a feminine journey in that it is circular; it spirals inward, and there are steps forward and then steps to the side or backward. The path meanders and moves not unlike a dance. But this dance is authentic and rhythmic and is led by the music of instinct and intuition.

I planted the seeds for my healing years before I returned to truly tend to them. It is deeply rewarding to connect with yourself, to tune in and settle into your spirit.

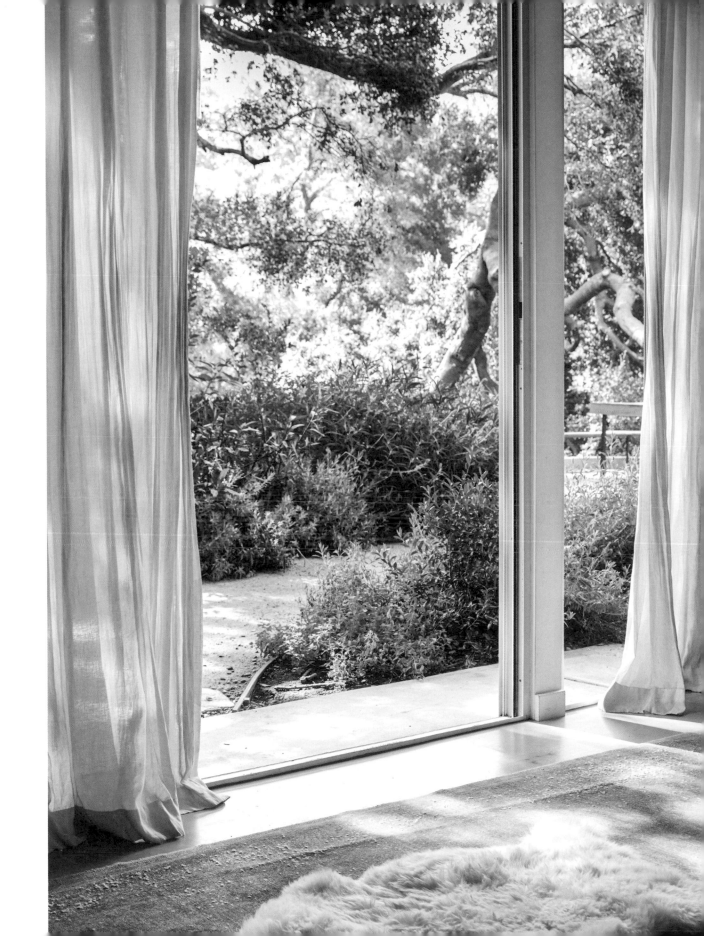

Introduction: My Whole Beauty Practices

As an active participant in the world of wellness, I speak only from my own experience. I want to share the touchstones that I return to again and again, which guide the information and approach in much of this book. But keep in mind, using your own creativity and intuition will no doubt turn your journey away from my path to one that is truly your own, and that's not only okay, but also a sign that you are following your heart to the place that is right for you.

Ritual

Ritual is at the heart of every aspect of this book, and it is the simplest and biggest way you can honor yourself and enhance your well-being. It is the difference between rushing through a shower or bath and consciously connecting with your body; between hastily splashing on body oil and taking the time to indulge your senses and anoint yourself; between speeding through your bedtime routine and savoring it with gratitude. Mindfulness and intention

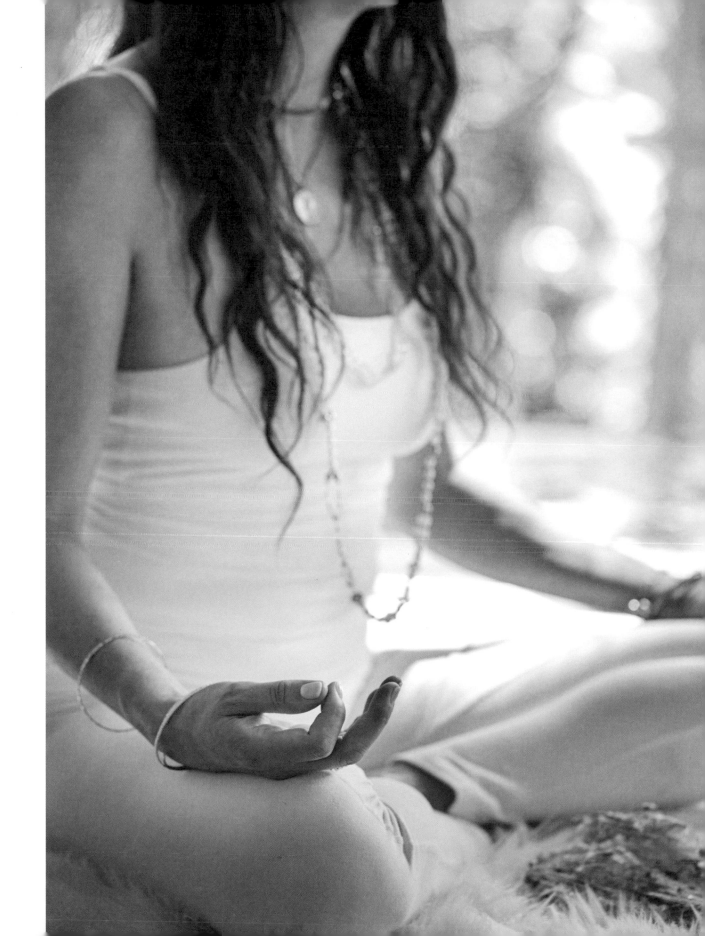

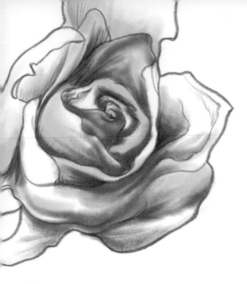

are the first steps in turning a routine into a ritual. They will transform self-care from a chore into an act of love. Creating rituals to acknowledge and induce pleasure is a form of religion, a way to care as much for the soul as for the skin. Beauty that does not penetrate beyond the first, physical layer will fade, but beauty that comes from being nourished and balanced spiritually, emotionally, and physically radiates from the eyes, hair, and every pore. Ritual helps us to create a beautiful face and a beautiful life.

Kundalini

Kundalini is a physical and spiritual practice. I did prenatal Kundalini when I was pregnant with my older daughter, but I began practicing regularly after going through my divorce. A friend who lived nearby was getting private lessons from Guru Jagat of the RA MA Institute in Venice, so I decided to try it three times a week, and I noticed profound shifts in my life. I then started to practice every day.

Kundalini combines yoga poses with meditations in the form of *kriya. Kriya* means "action," and it uses a series of postures, breath, and sound to trigger a physiological reaction in the brain that helps to change negative thought patterns to positive ones. Mantras can have the same effect through the use of sound. Kundalini employs mantras to "tune in" to the divine that is within all of us, and I frequently apply this same practice to my beauty rituals.

According to Yogi Bhajan, who is credited with bringing Kundalini to the United States, it is a "technology" that you can use to set change in motion. It replaces your old conditioning and generates self-love. Kundalini mantras, such as "I am bountiful, I am blissful, I am beautiful," resonate with people from all walks of life in their beauty and simplicity, and if you say those words often enough, you will start to believe them!

Ayurveda

Ayurveda is an Indian healing modality that is thousands of years old. In sharp contrast to Western medicine, in which only the symptoms of an illness or a disease are treated, Ayurveda is preventive, with the focus on constantly cleansing and detoxifying the body through practices like oil pulling (see page 115) and dry brushing (see page 116), and by following a holistic diet.

At the core of Ayurveda is the belief that people are made up of three life-giving forces, or doshas: Vata, Pitta, and Kapha.

The doshas are considered the inherent wisdom of the body and fuel the function of our bodies. When the three doshas are perfectly aligned, we are considered healthy. This doesn't necessarily mean the doshas are balanced equally. One of them is usually primary, another is secondary, and the third is the least influential. Everyone has a specific pattern of energy, which makes up his or her constitution, or *prakruti*.

Each dosha is made up of a combination of some of the five elements: air, water, earth, fire, and ether. According to Ayurveda, all health issues arise from an imbalance of the five elements. By balancing the doshas and their corresponding elements, you can alleviate most skin problems. This is typically done through diet and what you put on the skin, and by connecting the mind, body, and spirit. Most of us have all of the doshas, but to identify the prominent one, you can take self-assessment quizzes on Ayurvedic websites such as those of Banyan Botanicals or the Chopra Center, or see an Ayurvedic practitioner (you can find one through the National Ayurvedic Medical Association); there is also an abundance of information about Ayurveda in books and online (see Resources). The more you study, the more intuitive you will become and the more your body will guide you toward what it needs.

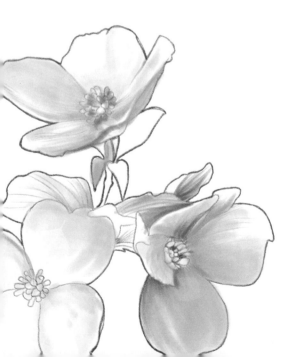

Vata

Vata is a combination of air and ether. This dosha promotes mobility, activity, and breath. When Vata is balanced, we can easily evoke joy, happiness, and lightness of being. When it's out of balance, we might feel fearful, anxious, and nervous. A person dominant in Vata will typically be underweight, with poor circulation and rough or dry skin. He or she will walk quickly, have a quick mind, and crave sweet and sour foods, like chocolate and lemons.

Pitta

Pitta is a combination of fire and water. This dosha controls our digestion, metabolism, and energy production. When Pitta is balanced, we are moving, thinking, and understanding things really quickly. When it's out of balance, we might experience frustration, anger, and argumentative behavior. A person dominant in Pitta will typically be of medium build, with a warm body temperature and oily skin. He or she will be a night owl, with intense cravings for greasy foods like pizza and French fries, and spicy foods, like hot sauce.

Kapha

Kapha is a combination of earth and water. This dosha is the energetic force behind the body's structure, what holds cells together and forms bone, muscle, fat, and sinew. With Kapha in balance, we feel harmonious, full of love, and calm. When it's out of balance, we'll often feel stubborn and resistant to change. A person dominant in Kapha might have a larger frame and be a bit heavier. He or she might feel sluggish and have a strong craving for sweets.

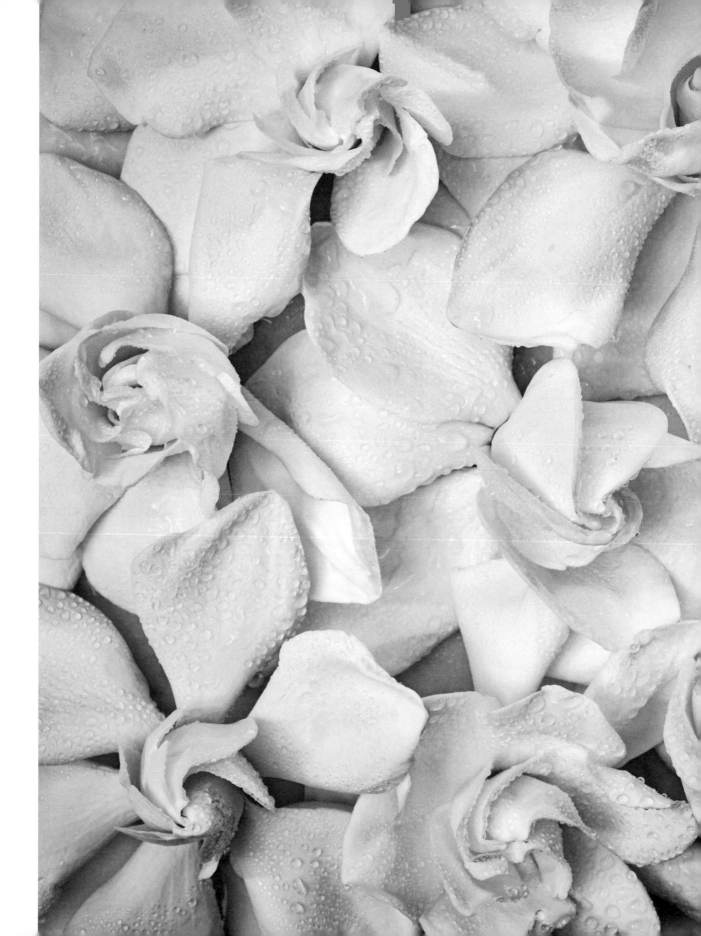

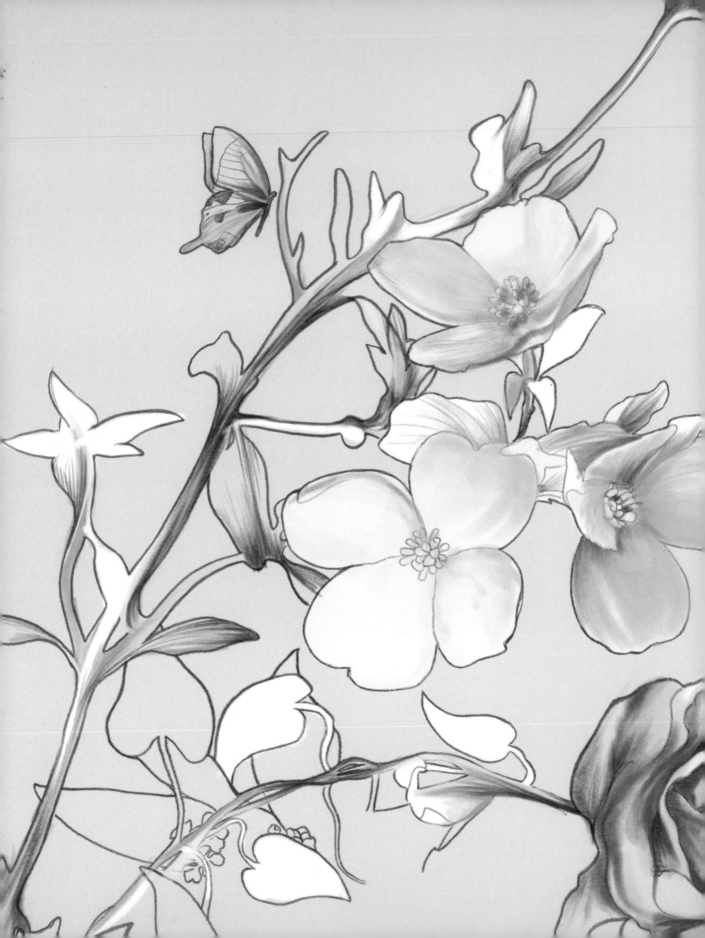

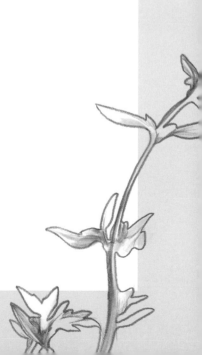

CHAPTER ONE

Making Space & Time for Daily Rituals

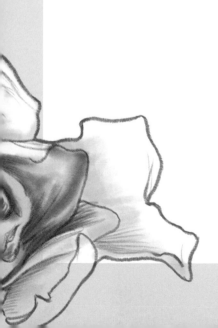

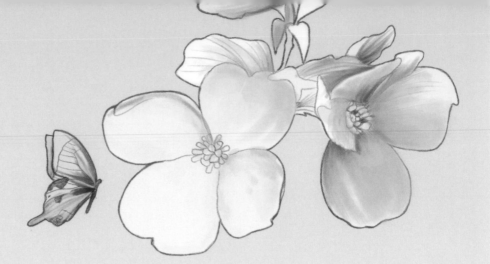

As women, we are inherently tribal. We are meant to gather with other women, to care for one another, participate in ceremony, and be in circles. Unfortunately, we often lack this connection in our modern lives, where we work in cubicles, frequently care for our families alone, and have mothers and sisters who live far away. Our days pass without a sense of reverence and community, and we're left with a powerful yearning for connection.

For me, rituals provide that connection. When I perform them alone, I am able to connect with the source of all being (our own, personal version of a higher power) and my deepest levels of self. When I gather for ceremony with other women, I connect with the divine feminine and form strong bonds with my teachers and friends, new sisters and mothers. Ritual and ceremony provide us with an opportunity to refuel, reenergize, and even reinvent ourselves. Just a simple beauty ritual can trigger a profound shift into a more self-healing modality.

I experienced my first ritual almost two decades ago, and it really enlightened me and opened me up to a whole new realm of healing. I was in Santa Fe, New Mexico, with my family, and it was the middle of winter. In the coldest months, New Mexico is a magical, mystical place, with its dusty, red landscape awash in drifts of white snow. My former mother-in-law and I traveled to a small adobe house on the outskirts of town, where a Native American shaman held ceremonies in her sweat lodge.

This was my introduction to the use of cleansing herbs, such as sage, and to the power of prayer. The lodge was the hottest place I had ever been, and we were naked for the three-hour ceremony. It was a test of strength, will, and spirit. I openly cried as the chants and smoke and sweat unearthed the demons I thought I had so carefully buried. There were many moments when I wanted to leave, but even when my mind told me I wouldn't last a minute longer, my spirit told me to stay.

In these moments, I would lower myself to the ground and put my naked breasts against the cool earth. I felt the feminine power of the earth supporting me. As I breathed in the cool air that rose up to revive me, I knew that if I could survive this, I could survive anything outside of the lodge as well.

After the sweat, I emerged renewed, and my senses were alive. I saw rainbows and shimmering orbs. The shaman had laid out a beautiful feast of hummus, crackers, olives, salads, and fresh juices, and all the food glittered like gems. Everything tasted incredible, and I felt like I had been stripped raw to reignite my passion for beauty and pleasure.

During this ritual, the shaman told me that I was connected to the wolf, and she used the word *lupus*, which is the Latin translation. This was my first inkling of my autoimmune disorders, and I would be formally diagnosed with lupus a short while later.

I don't think we have to go to this extreme to have ritual in our lives. That just happened to be my initiation into this newfound world. When I come together with my sisters, most of the rituals we perform are very simple. We will gather flowers, make a mandala, and call in the Four Directions, which is a Native American tradition that represents a universal way of connecting with the earth. For a small ritual, often with just one other person, a tea ceremony connects us to nature and roots us in the moment. Something as simple as lighting a candle and saying a prayer can take ordinary life and elevate it to a higher realm.

The most important thing is how you approach what you are doing. Mindfulness and intention are the only requirements for turning a routine into a ritual. Are you approaching your beauty treatments as a chore or as an act of self-love? Are you distractedly slathering on body oil or taking the time to anoint yourself?

In a world that dulls the senses with overstimulation and overextension, women are losing touch with their desire and need for pleasure. As a result, we are starving for these very things. We need to be illuminated and filled up by the divine, and we can do this by creating moments of happiness and abundance in our lives.

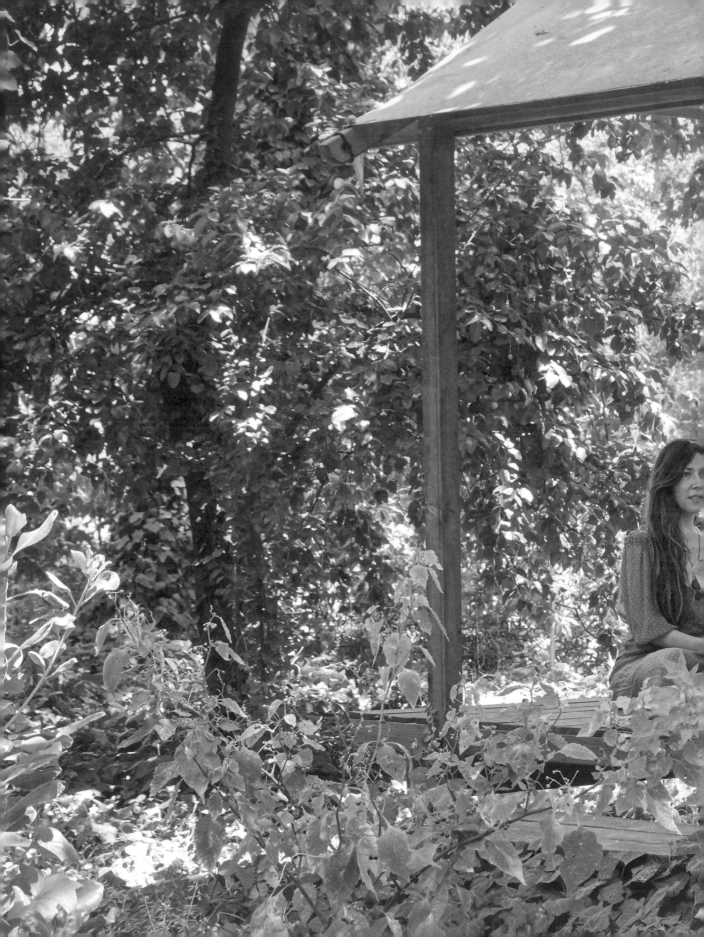

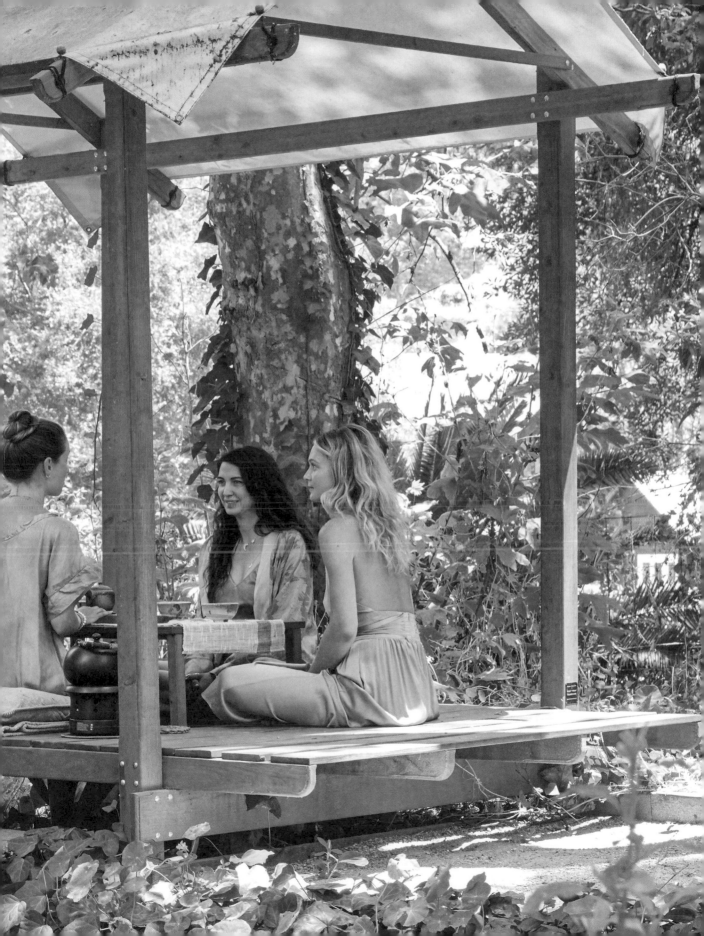

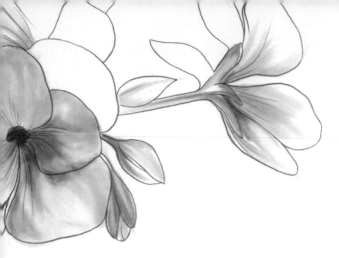

Creating a Sacred Space

The temples on either side of the forehead are reminders that we can create temples (sacred places) wherever we go just by closing our eyes and imagining them—no money or design experience needed. However, I do think that actually creating a sacred space in your home can make you feel closer to the rituals and awaken your desire to do more. Your sacred space can be a whole room or a tiny altar on a table, but it will become the place where you apply your beauty masks, meditate, do yoga, read cards, write in your journal, or set intentions for the new moon.

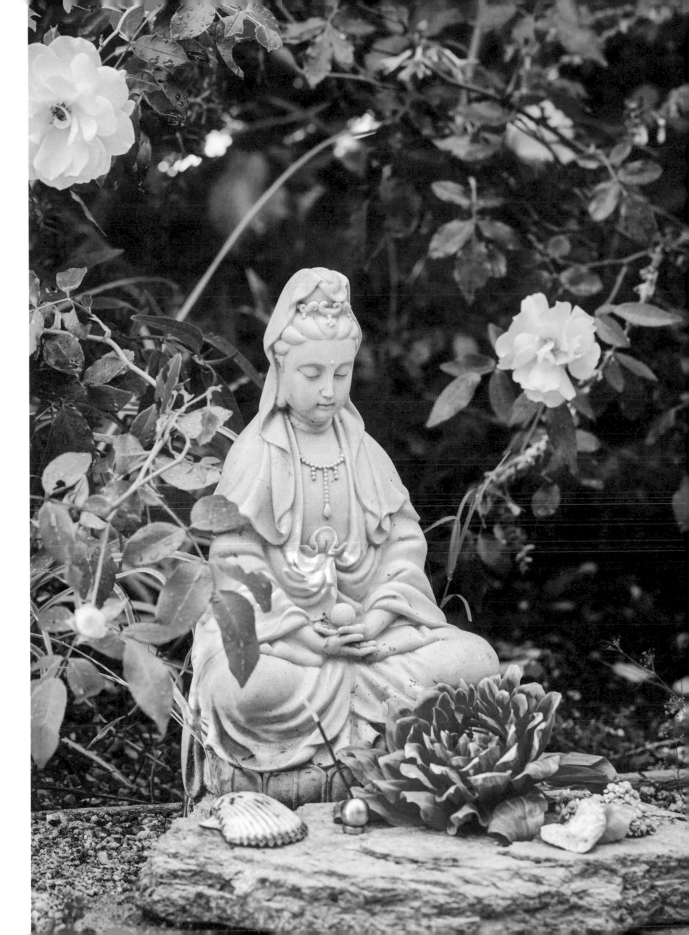

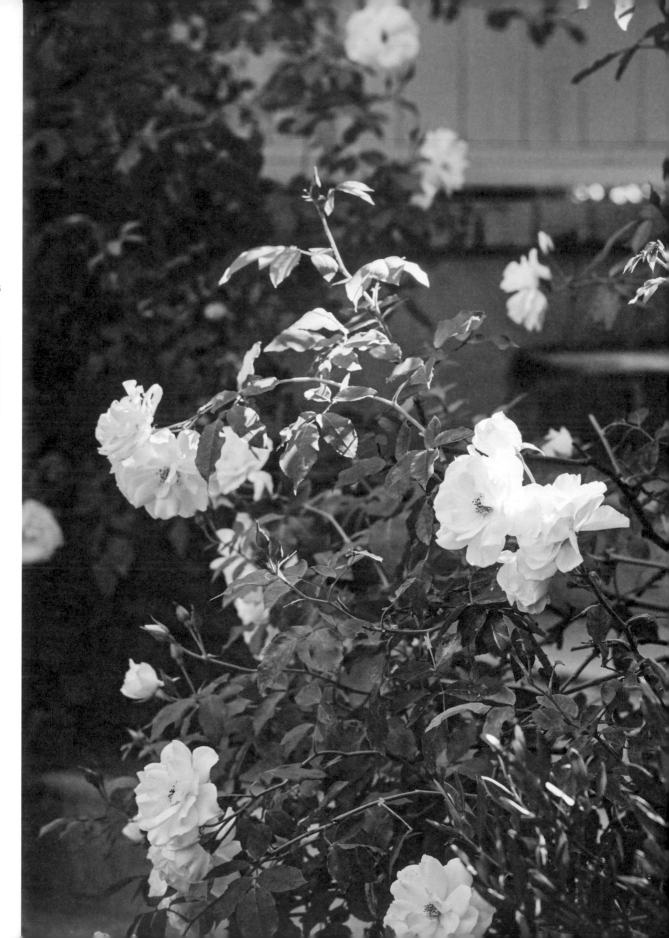

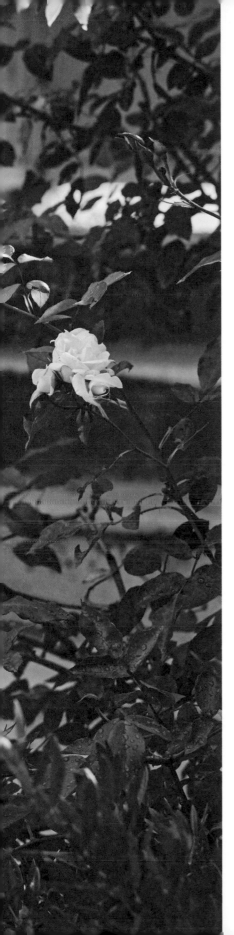

It is the place where we go to connect to the source of all being and hone our intuition. As women, we're inclined to create atmosphere, we're inclined to create beauty around us, we're inclined toward being sensitive to our environment, and altars are a beautiful way to honor these inclinations.

Altars represent your life. When you clean the altar, you can imagine you're cleaning your life. When you offer flowers, or fruit, or incense, you're offering those to your life. Anything you do for the altar is also a meditation and intention for your life.

I personally have a few different altars. I have a nature altar, which is where I keep my crystals and things from the natural world. My children and I will add flowers in the springtime, seashells in the summer, fallen leaves in autumn, and pinecones in the winter. I have an altar to my womb, which is just a very simple space on the floor with a candle, a big rose quartz, and a beautiful piece of silk fabric. I'll light incense there, and this is where I'll sit to do my yoni egg exercises (see page 98). I have an altar for mother energy and the sacred feminine, and an altar where I practice Nichiren Buddhism. Altars don't have to cost a lot to make, but they embody the idea of creating a sacred space that's just for you. An altar alters you. Virginia Woolf is famous for saying that every woman needs a room of her own, and I think we can take that sentiment and say that every woman needs an altar of her own.

Making Your Own Altar

Your altar can be as malleable and ever-changing as you are. You are not always in the same mood, dealing with the same difficulties, or pursuing the same goals, so you can adapt your altar to reflect whatever you need to honor or bring into your life at that specific point in time. There is no right or wrong way to build an altar, and the best way to do it is to let your intention guide you. You may include any or all of the following and more.

- Crystals
- Flowers
- Pictures of loved ones
- Images of goddesses
- Family mementos (like a beloved relative's jewelry, or something made by your children)
- Things found in nature (rocks, feathers, shells, sticks)
- A bowl of coins (for abundance)
- Incense
- Essential oils
- A mirror (helpful for doing beauty rituals in front of the altar)
- Candles (I choose the color depending on what emotion I want to bring in, a practice I've adopted from Wiccan literature; see the list at right)

CANDLE COLORS AND THEIR MEANINGS

PINK
Love

YELLOW
Clarity

PURPLE
Intuition

GREEN
Prosperity

BLUE
Peace and Healing

RED
Passion

WHITE
Blessings

BLACK
Removing Negativity

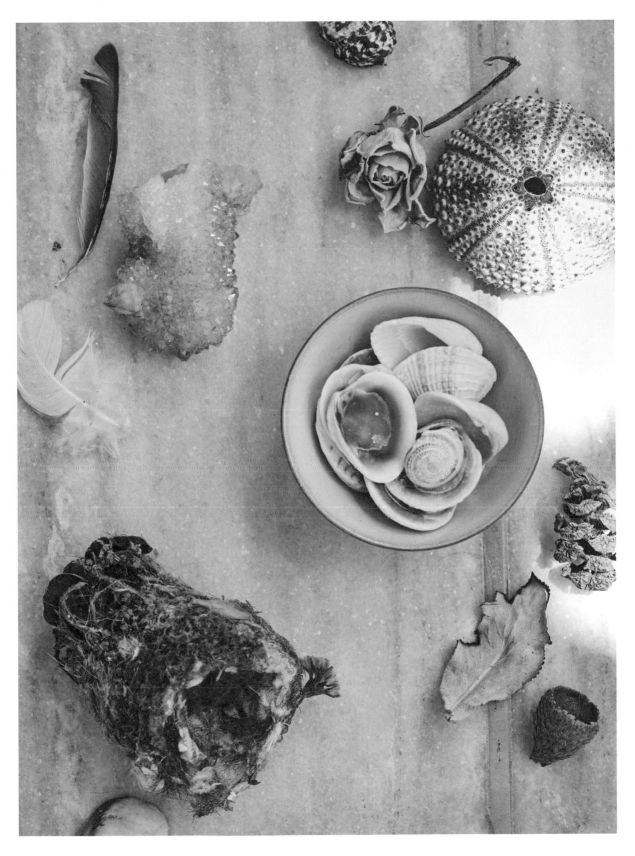

Space Clearing

When I got divorced, one of the things that was most upsetting was knowing that my daughters and I would have to leave the beautiful 1914 Mission-style house that we loved and called home.

What got me through that time was imagining what I wanted in my life. I couldn't quite see the style of the house we would live in, but I did imagine a glass wall of green—as if we could look out into a forest of some kind—and lots of light. A friend of mine kept referring to this feeling as "the call of the wild." I also needed to feel content and connected to our new home, feelings I'd experienced over the years and wanted to experience again.

After a year of looking, our time was running out. One day I saw a house that wasn't very suitable but had wonderful trees. When I first walked in, I was instantly charmed by the couple selling it, who had been married for almost half a century and were still very much in love. They'd built the house in 1949 and though it was dilapidated, the caring energy within it was palpable. As I moved from room to room, it grew increasingly clear that renovating the place would pose an enormous challenge. However, when I went outside into the garden and took in the majestic oaks, I began to cry. I knew the trees had drawn me there. I had to quiet my racing mind (*The cost to restore this house will be too much.*

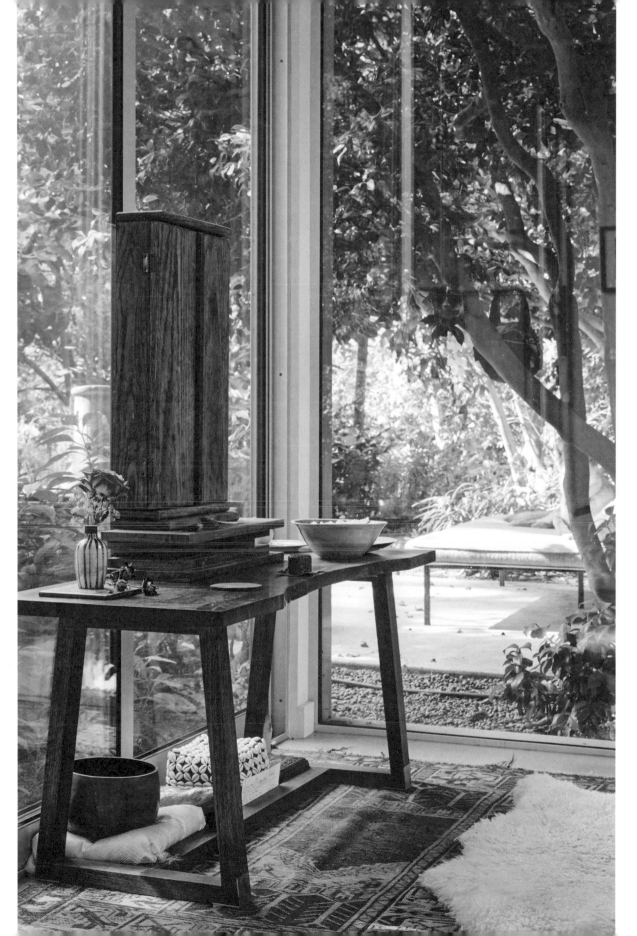

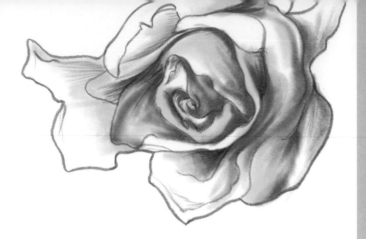

It needs a new roof. The carpets are stained with dog urine. What about the electrical wiring?) and listen to my gut, my heart, and my spirit. The energy of the house called to me, and said, "This is home. You are home." I feel so grateful that I listened to my intuition rather than my pragmatism or ego.

The more you tune in to yourself and your own energy, the more sensitive you will become to the energy of places and other people. Whenever I come into a new space, I like to clear the energy from the past and set the stage for new blessings.

Thousands of years ago, people didn't believe in bacteria because they couldn't see it. I like to use that metaphor to describe energy. Just because we can't see energy doesn't mean it isn't there.

Clearing a space of previous energy is very meditative and a way of hitting reset on your mind, heart, and space, reminding them to stay open so that you can receive new blessings. Following are a few of my favorite ways to clear space.

Sage

Sage is one of the many reasons I feel so blessed to call California home. Here, this wonderful medicinal plant grows wild on hiking trails. It is easy for me to pick enough to bundle or just snap off a few fragrant leaves to crush in my hands as I walk.

A PRAYER TO
ACCOMPANY SMUDGING

May your hands be
cleansed, that they might
create beautiful things.

May your feet be cleansed,
that they might take you
where you most need to be.

May your heart be cleansed,
that you might hear its
messages clearly.

May your throat be cleansed,
that you might speak rightly
when words are needed.

May your eyes be cleansed,
that you might see the signs
and wonders of the world.

May this person and space be
washed clean by the smoke
of these fragrant plants.

And may that same smoke
carry your prayers,
spiraling, to the heavens.

The burning of sage is most often associated with Native Americans, who performed ceremonial smudging to rid spaces and people of negative energy, dispel illness, and set the stage for new beginnings and good fortune.

If, like me, you live someplace where it is easy to find wild sage, you can make your own smudge wand by binding several stems together with string and hanging it upside down to dry out. You can also dry out and burn individual leaves.

Sage bundles are also easy to find at metaphysical shops, health food stores, and small gift and home shops. (I sell them in my online store as well.) White sage is the type most commonly used in smudging, and you'll often find it mixed with other herbs, like sweet grass for positive energy and juniper or cedar for healing.

Burn your sage in a heatproof container to catch all the ash and embers. An abalone shell is traditional, but you can also use a copper bowl, a terra-cotta pot, or any other vessel that is safe and also pleasing to you.

Light the sage, and when it goes out (you may have to blow on it) and starts to smoke, use your hand or a feather or another lightweight object to disperse the smoke into all four corners of the room and around your altar while imagining all of the energy of the past being carried away with the drifting smoke. Make sure all the doors and windows are open.

You can also burn sage when recovering from an illness, after an argument with your significant other, or any time you feel the need to refresh and reset your environment. You can smudge people too, by sweeping the smoke along their limbs, across their body, and under their feet.

I like to accompany the act of smudging with the Native American prayer opposite.

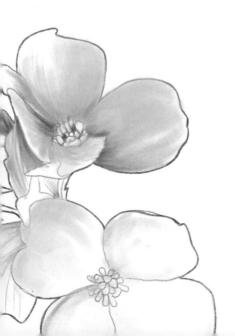

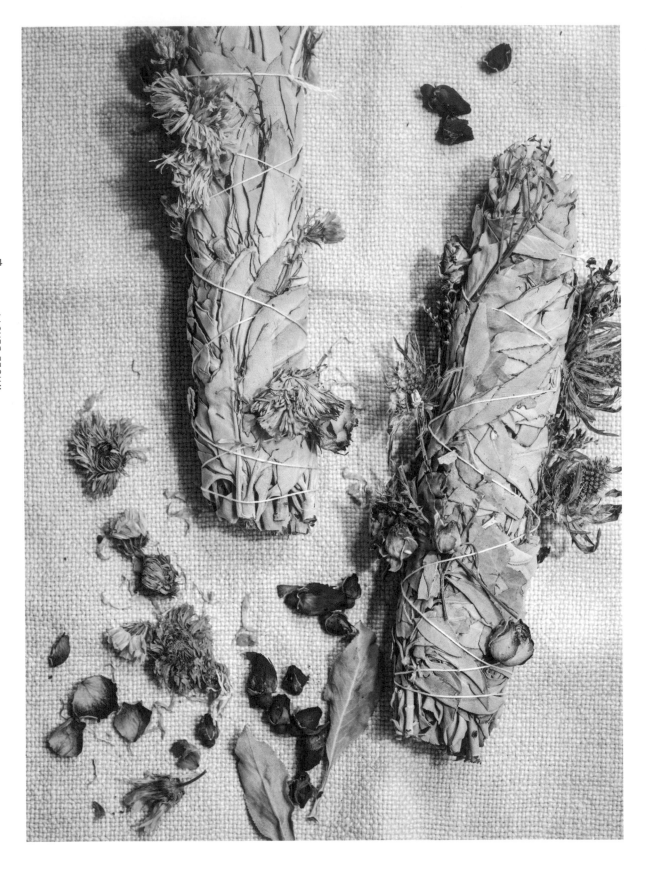

Salt

If you have ever been to a healer and noticed a bowl of salt in the corner of the room, it probably wasn't there to spice up his or her lunch. Salt is renowned for its ability to absorb and trap negative energy that is released from people, objects, and events.

The easiest way to clear a space with salt is to place small bowls in each corner of the room, mindfully stating your intention as you do so. I like to say, "I cleanse this room of any impurities, negativity, or anything that doesn't support my highest good. Amen." Leave the salt for twenty-four hours, then discard it. I like to do this whenever I move into a new home, before rituals or tea ceremonies, or after any stressful situation in the home, and then I bury the salt or throw it into the ocean.

Incense

The burning of incense as part of ceremony and ritual is something that you will find across cultures and religions. In Buddhist temples, circular coils of incense are burned to bring forth bodhisattvas and other deities. In Christian and Jewish ceremonies, incense is lit so that the burning smoke may represent the prayers of the faithful rising to heaven. In Hinduism, incense is often a daily offering to a god, and on a Wiccan altar, a lit stick of incense represents the element of air.

Incense was often crafted from whatever materials were available locally, like wood, bark, flowers, resin, or roots, so the types of incense used during rituals differed greatly from region to region.

Use any type of nontoxic incense that is pleasing to you in form and scent. After cleansing, the burning of incense welcomes in angels, ancestors, and spirits to bring blessings and guide you on your way.

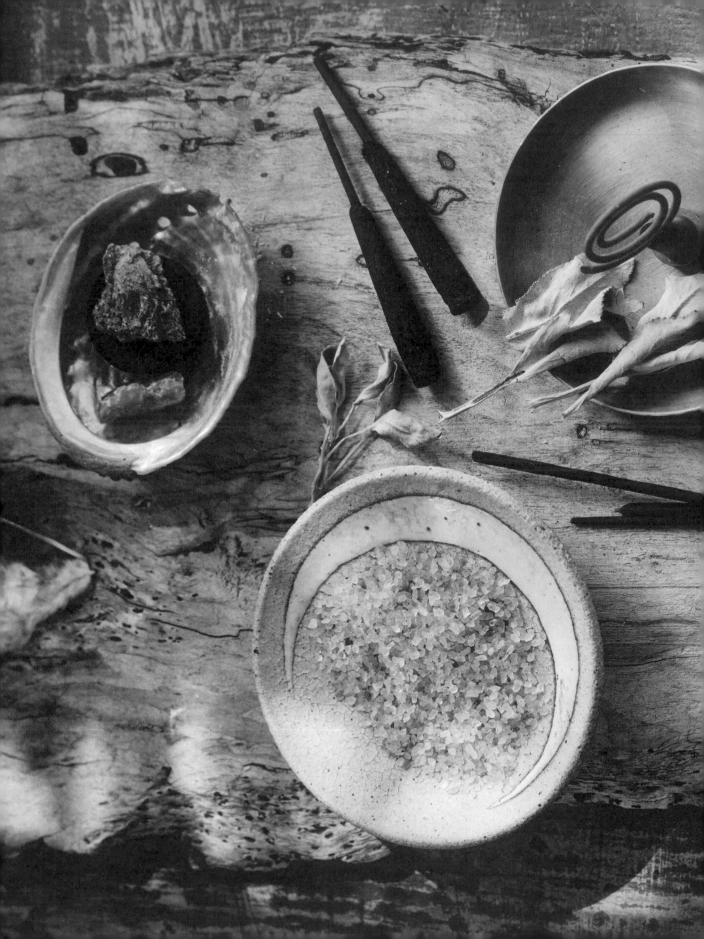

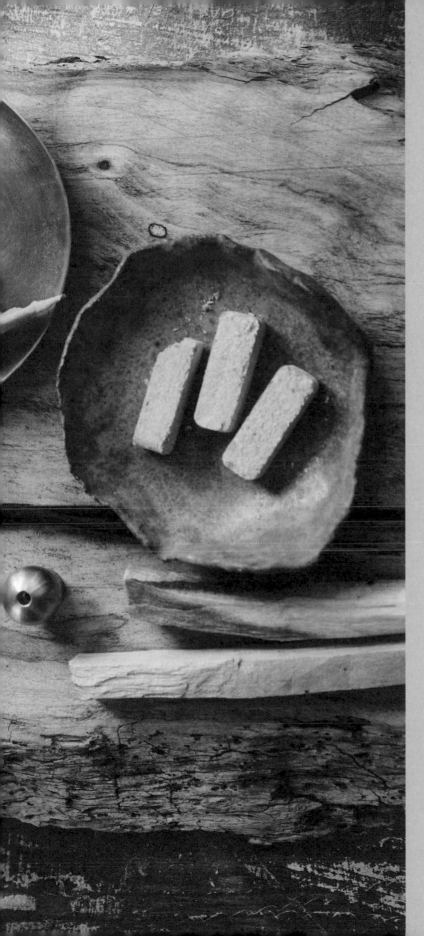

MY FAVORITE INCENSES

Cedar or Pine
These woodsy scents smell
clean and fresh, and they
clear negative energy.

Copal
Smoky and lush, copal powerfully
cleanses spaces and auras.

Frankincense
This sweet scent is used for
purification and heightened
spirituality. It traditionally
represents masculine energy.

Myrrh
An earthy, almost anise
scent that is used to bring
in positive energy, myrrh
traditionally is seen as a
representation of feminine energy.
Frankincense and myrrh are often
burned or blended together,
since they represent a balance.

New Mexico Piñon
This incense is made from
an evergreen tree that grows
in New Mexico, Arizona, Texas,
and Wyoming. When burned,
it has a beautiful woodsy scent.
It was traditionally lit during
a Native American ceremony
for protection. Prayers can
be sent through the smoke.

Calling in the Four Directions

For bigger rituals, like a circle with friends, celebrating the new or full moon with my sisters, or the beginning of a retreat, I will call in the Four Directions. This is a Native American prayer that honors the elements and pays homage to the belief that all life is interconnected. We humans are an integral part of nature, so every time we honor Mother Earth, we are also honoring ourselves. I particularly enjoy this prayer because it links me to my Native American ancestors. I begin by facing east, then turn my body ninety degrees with each new verse, completely opening the space so that the divine force may enter it to bless us.

A Prayer to Call in the Four Directions

Great spirits of the east, the land of the rising sun, the land of new beginnings and birth of beginnings. The land of the great condor and the eagle, please join me here today in this sacred space. Please bring me your energy, please protect me under your wings as the great condor does. Please let me see the great perspective of my life from the heights of the eagle and the condor. Thank you for being here today, great spirits of the east.

Great spirits of the south, the land of fire, the land of ambition, the land of desire, sexuality, fertility. Thank you for being here today with me. The land of the great serpent, please allow me to shed what no longer serves me, as a snake does. Please allow the coils of the light and the coils of protection to surround me here today. Great spirits of the south, please ignite my passion and my ambition for the betterment of this planet. Thank you, great spirits of the south.

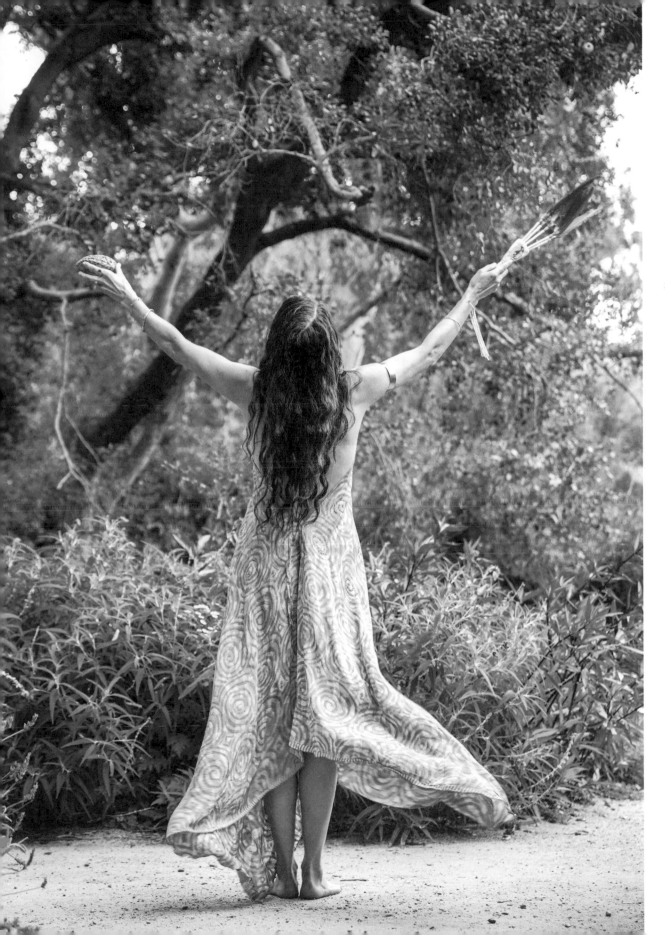

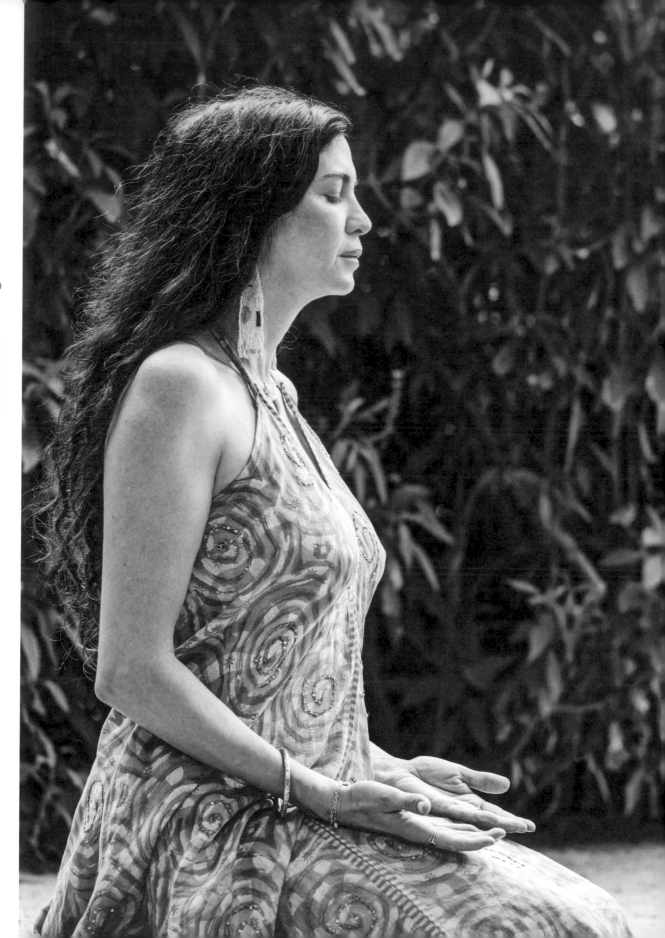

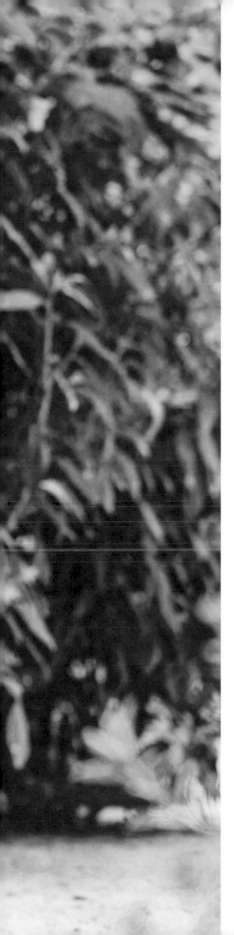

Great spirits of the west, the land of the setting sun. The land of dreams, the land of the unconscious, the land of water, thank you for being here today with me. I want to give a blessing of gratitude for all the rains you have brought us. I would like to honor all the ways in which water blesses my life. The land of the jaguar, the land of medicine, please be here with me today. Thank you, great spirits of the west.

Great spirits of the north, the land of the ancestors. Thank you for all my ancestors, seven generations past. Thank you for protecting me, and for the seven generations to come. Thank you for being here today, hummingbird medicine, bear medicine, all that come from the north. Let me be able to take in the sweet nectar of my life, as the hummingbird takes in nectar from the flowers around. Let me have the strength and wisdom of the bear. Thank you, great winds and spirits of the north.

Great Mama Earth, Pachamama, Gaia, thank you for being here today with me. Thank you for all your blessings, thank you for the mountains, the rivers, the streams, the creeks. Thank you for all your creatures, the two-legged, the four-legged, the creepy-crawlies, the winged ones, the finned ones. Thank you. Thank you for protecting us. I offer to be a guardian for you. I offer to bring you protection. Thank you for being here today with me, O great spirit of Mother Earth.

Great spirits of the sky, celestial beings, Father Sky, Mother Moon, Sister Wind, Star Nation People, thank you for all your energy. Thank you for shining your light among us. Thank you for being here today with me.

At the end of the ritual, it is important to close the space, so I like to conclude with something very simple:

Thank you for being with us today, great spirits of the east, great spirits of the south, great spirits of the west, great spirits of the north, and the celestial mothers and fathers. Thank you.

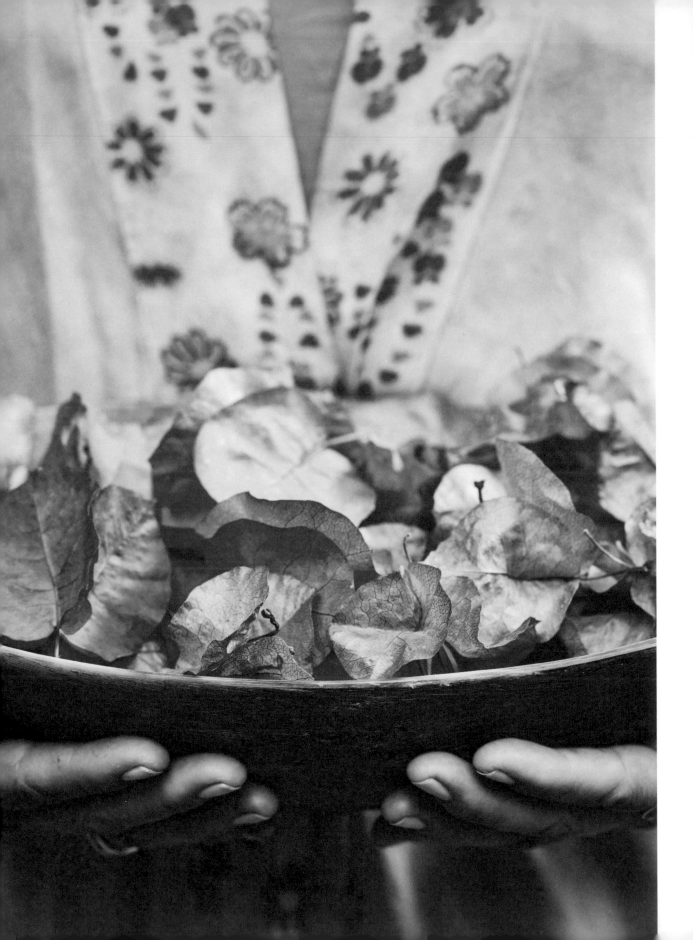

A Simple Ritual Opening

Sometimes we don't have the time or space for a full ritual but still want to honor something with an intention. In those moments, I like to use these simple words to bring mindfulness and awareness to my beauty rituals and practices.

I am now connecting to the source, the source of all being, and I'm asking that my heart be open for this ritual that I'm about to begin. I want to thank all my guides that watch over me and all the earth's energy that watches over me. I want to be able to fill myself with love and abundance and the light of the universe. I am bountiful, I am blissful, I am beautiful.

Goddesses

I have always called myself a feminine feminist, a phrase Anaïs Nin coined so perfectly. I love using the feminine within me to bring more power and sensuality to women everywhere. Women today live in the masculine energy more than ever, and we are now the providers in so many ways. This can be fulfilling, yet exhausting. Bringing the goddess energy into our lives helps us to balance ourselves and the world around us. The more we become familiar with the goddesses, the more we learn to recognize and acknowledge them.

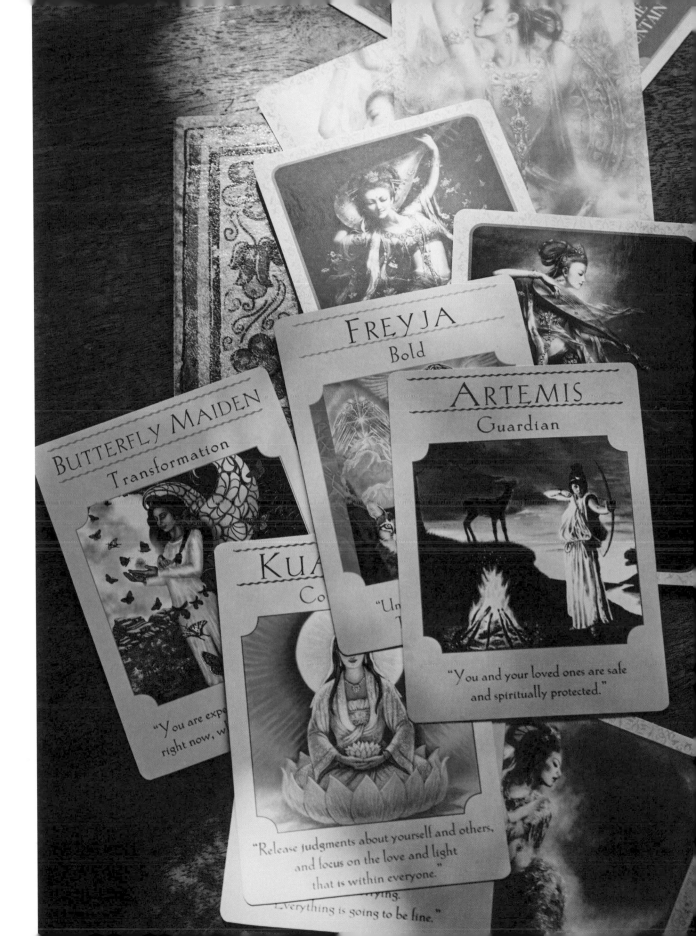

The goddesses help us to break out of a rut we may be stuck in and celebrate other aspects of who we are, honoring all the dimensions of our lives.

Lately, I feel like I am dating the different goddesses—taking them each out for a night or two to experience the unique qualities and characteristics they have to offer.

Working with a goddess is developing a personal relationship with her and learning to approach and honor her in a way that feels individual and true to you. On the following pages are examples of how I speak to and call my favorite goddesses, but as with all ritual, the power here is in the intention. You do not need to follow these guidelines explicitly, as long as your intention is clear and you are working from a mindful, heartfelt place. Feel free to alter the prayers. The objects are suggestions of what to add to your altar to call in each particular goddess, but again, you may use whatever is most sacred to you.

A note on chakras as they relate to the goddesses: Chakra *means "wheel" in Sanskrit, and the chakras are the seven turning wheels of our energy field (or subtle body). The chakras can be found from the top of the head down to the bottom of the spine. When they are active and spinning, they brighten our aura. When they are closed and stagnant, our aura dims. When our chakras are balanced and working together, we feel confident, calm, and energized, both grounded and in touch with our divine self. For more about chakras, see pages 83–86.*

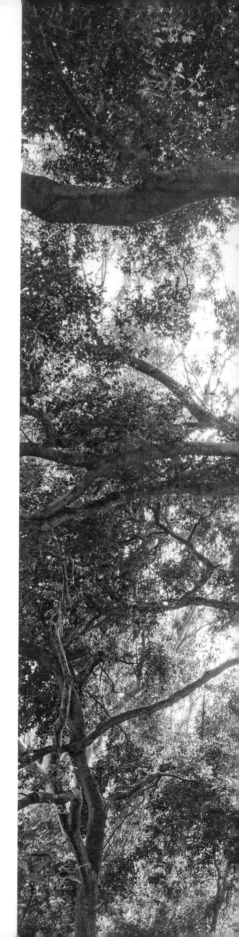

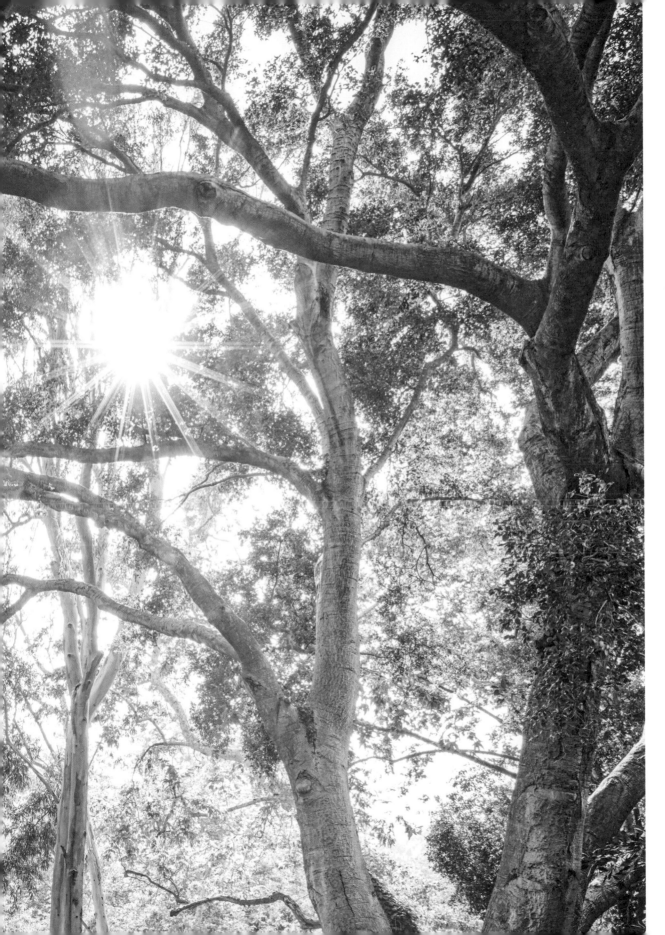

MAKING SPACE & TIME FOR DAILY RITUALS

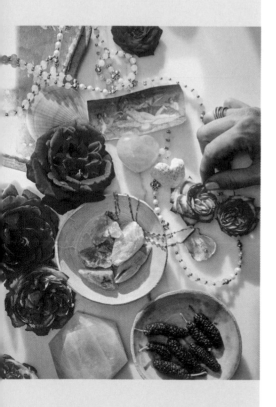

Venus

Venus (or Aphrodite in ancient Greece) is the ancient Roman goddess of love, sex, fertility, abundance, and harvest. I have felt a kinship to her for some time now, and every morning in my meditation I acknowledge this presence in my life. When you honor Venus, you are evoking the feminine, the fertile, and the forces of beauty, compassion, and love. You can bring out the Venus in you when you nourish yourself. Venus can give us the courage to be bolder and to stand in our light, acknowledging our radiance and power.

Venus came from the sea and was born in water. Every year in ancient Rome, on the first day of April, women lowered the statue of Venus and ritually bathed her in honor of feminine sexuality and sensuality. So one way to acknowledge Venus and this ancient ritual is with a bath. Add rose petals and rose essential oils, or go bathe in a lake or the ocean. Make a flower mandala or a seashell design in your garden or somewhere else in the natural world. Venus reminds you to treat yourself the way you want to be treated by others.

A Prayer for Venus

Dear Venus, I am calling upon you to join me here today. I am calling upon your shining starlight to open my crown chakra and breathe love into my heart. I ask for your guidance in bringing me closer to loved ones and healing myself from past wounds. I ask that I use your pink-white energy to bring beauty to all I do. I ask that I can bring healing through my work and a celebration of all that is you.

Sacred Objects for Venus

Red roses, mirrors, rose quartz, luscious fruit, chocolates, milk, honey. Images of Venus by the old masters. Seashells and pearls. Things that bring you joy.

Parvati

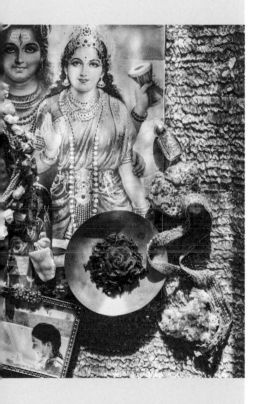

Parvati is the Hindu goddess of love, seduction, and luminosity. She's a truth seeker, a mother, and wife to Shiva, the god of the yogis. She's one of my favorites because she's very romantic. When she fell in love with Shiva, he wanted nothing to do with her, yet she waited for him until he changed his mind. She never gave up, and in the end, they became a powerful couple who changed the world with their deep love.

Call on Parvati to enhance your relationship, to summon your future love, and to bring protection to your home and family. She embodies kindness, grace, and strength and is a reminder to women that we can be strong and feminine at the same time.

A Prayer for Parvati

Dear Parvati, I call upon your divine energy to bless my home, my family, and my beloved. I call upon your gracious nature to imbue my workspace and all my creations with your honor and blessings. Nurture me so that I may be able to nurture my children and my beloved. Allow me to have your grace, patience, focus, and open and loving heart in all matters of love in my life.

Sacred Objects for Parvati

Think of Parvati as a queen, and make your offerings accordingly: fruit, incense, gold, amethyst, crowns, pictures of your children, rubies, aquamarine, hibiscus flowers.

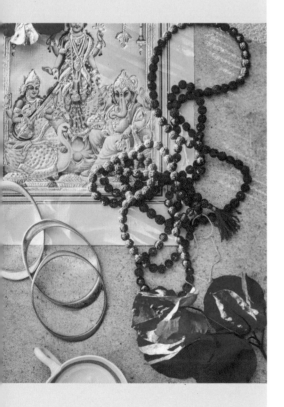

Lakshmi

Lakshmi is the Hindu goddess of fortune and beauty. Like Venus, she came from the sea. When she was born, she emerged fully grown on a pink lotus flower rising up from the water. Lakshmi is a powerful ally to call on to help fulfill professional aspirations, including achieving financial success. She inspires confidence, because confidence leads to abundance. She is a peacemaker and the goddess of working mothers. She's also attracted to cleanliness, so it's good to tidy up your workspace so that she will be drawn in. I generally do a good cleaning on the new moon (for new beginnings). Lakshmi loves music, so another way to honor her is to put some on and sing or dance! *Shanti* means "peace," and "Shanti shanti shanti" is one of her mantras.

A Prayer for Lakshmi
Dear Lakshmi, I call upon you today and ask that you guide me with your wisdom. Allow me to bring more abundance and blessings into my world so that I can help myself and others. Allow me to feel deserving of success and bounty. Allow me to use my good fortune for the betterment of my community and planet.

Sacred Objects for Lakshmi
A beautiful shawl, pink or red flowers, gold coins, lotus flowers, jewelry, fans. Clean your house in her honor, and put a picture of her above the stove so that the heat can activate her powers.

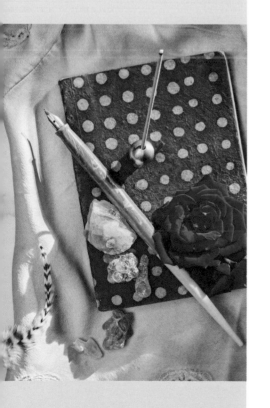

Freyja

Freyja is the Norse goddess of love and fertility. She's one of the most powerful deities and can aid in healing past traumas. She's very sensual and can bring sexuality and wildness into your life. She is seen with wings or wearing feathers and is represented by birds of prey like hawks, falcons, and eagles. I am always inspired by Freyja because she is unafraid of her sexuality. She will help you to become more magnetic, own your energy, and ignite fires in your lower chakras.

A Prayer for Freyja

Dear Freyja, please allow me to ignite my sexual identity and my sexual power. Please allow me to heal any past wounds that are keeping me from fulfilling my desires. Allow me to connect to my internal fire and to awaken my lower chakras.

Sacred Objects for Freyja

Take out a pen and write a list of things you wish to attract. Light a candle to symbolize Freyja's flame, and place the list and a piece of beautiful lingerie on your altar. Anoint your altar with the scent of musk or amber. Put on some music that will make you dance with abandon. Go on arduous hikes in the wild and bring home a beautiful rock that symbolizes strength.

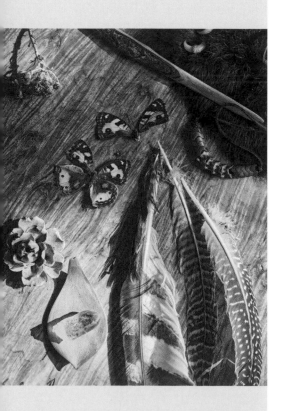

Artemis

Artemis (Diana in ancient Rome) is the ancient Greek goddess of the hunt and embodies independence and passion. She can help you advance in your career and pursue new opportunities. She has a laser focus and does not apologize for being self-reliant. I like to think of her as the lady of the wild things, spending her days in the forest with her posse of animals. She is often pictured with a bow and arrow.

Summon the spirit of Artemis when you are in need of more power and strength. Call upon her when you need a guardian to protect you. She is also of service when you need to summon your strength for heading into battle, or even childbirth.

A Prayer for Artemis

Dear Artemis, please allow me to have more focus, determination, and drive. Allow my ambition to benefit my life and to better the planet. Please give me your wisdom and your tools so that I may accomplish my goals. Allow me to hone my animal-like instincts to strengthen my intuitive powers.

Sacred Objects for Artemis

Found items from nature, like leaves, sticks, rocks, and feathers. Fire (like a candle or a fire you build in her honor in the fireplace). Arrowheads, arrows, butterflies, insect wings, bones, teeth, animal skins, pictures of beloved pets.

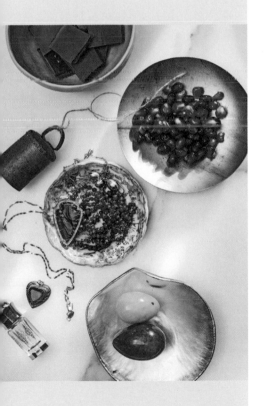

Lalita

Lalita is a yogic goddess who is all about flirtation, sensuality, and childlike fun. She reminds us that life should include lots of laughter and love. Lalita is also known for her beautiful dark hair, so summon her during hair treatments. She brings confidence and a sense of adventure, and she activates the erotic, so call on Lalita during your yoni egg exercises.

A Prayer for Lalita

Dear Lalita, goddess of desire, please magnetize my erotic feminine nature. Please bestow your energy on me and help me activate my sensuality and joy. Send me your wisdom and compassion regarding matters of the heart. Allow me to bring healing through love and my sensual nature.

Sacred Objects for Lalita

Perfume, pomegranates, berries, rubies, bells, arrows, some lubricant or body oil, yoni eggs, chocolate, an image of your lover. Or put on some music that creates an atmosphere you feel vibrant in. Do a dance just for yourself, or massage your beloved in her honor.

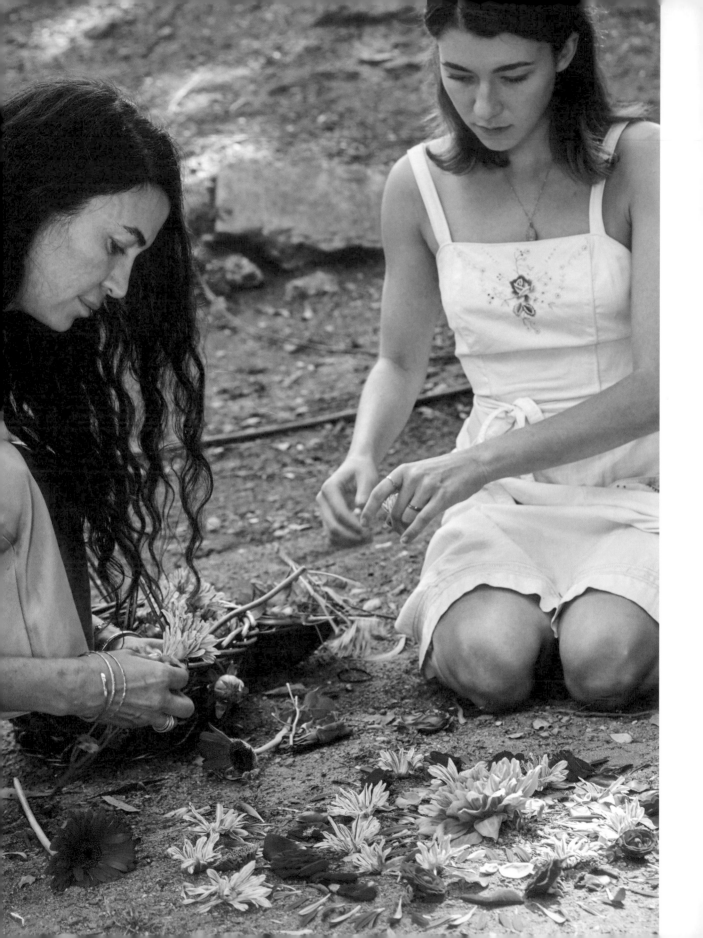

Honoring Nature with Ritual

Women have their own cycles and are very connected to the cycles of nature as well. I have a nature altar in my home that changes as the seasons change. When we go on walks, my daughters and I will bring home things to put on our altar. In the fall, these may be acorns or pinecones; in the springtime, blossoms or seeds. We'll add driftwood, seashells, and rocks—one of my most precious possessions is my collection of heart-shaped rocks! We also like to honor the changing seasons with rituals that remind us to care for the earth as we care for ourselves.

Spring

Spring is all about regrowth, renewal, and rebirth. This is the time of year when the world explodes with the scent and color of flowers. When I am hiking, or at home in my garden, I like to imprint this beauty on my soul by laying out a mandala of petals, sticks, leaves, rocks, and whatever else may be easily accessible. It is a very meditative practice that urges us to slow down and drink in all the beauty that surrounds us. The mandala can be shaped like a star, heart, flower, or design of your choosing. Let your creativity flow, and you will soon find that you are concentrating not on the trivial to-dos of the day but on the shapes, colors, and textures of nature.

Norooz, the Persian New Year, is celebrated on the spring equinox with a picnic outdoors by a river or spring. You can adapt this tradition by applying a beauty mask (there are many recipes in chapter 4) to help you shed your winter skin and embrace the healing of fresh, new beginnings.

Summer

Summer is a time to express gratitude and pay homage to all that you have harvested. Feast on cool, juicy fruits. Whenever you can, sit by still water to meditate (even a pool will do!). Since your skin is likely to be dehydrated from the sun and the heat, do what you can to replenish moisture. Break out your hydrosols (see page 265) and mist yourself throughout the day, expressing reverence for the water each time you do.

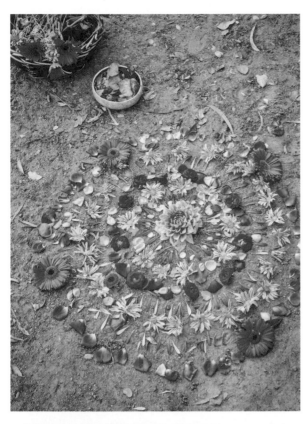

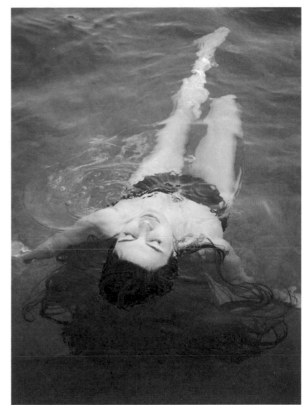

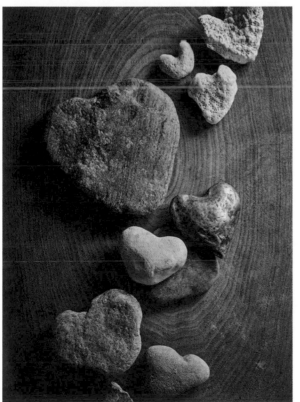

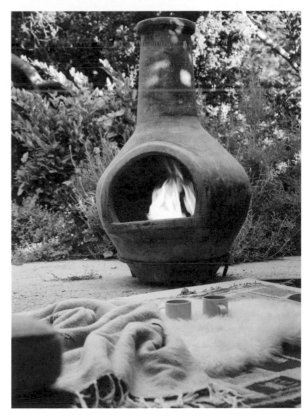

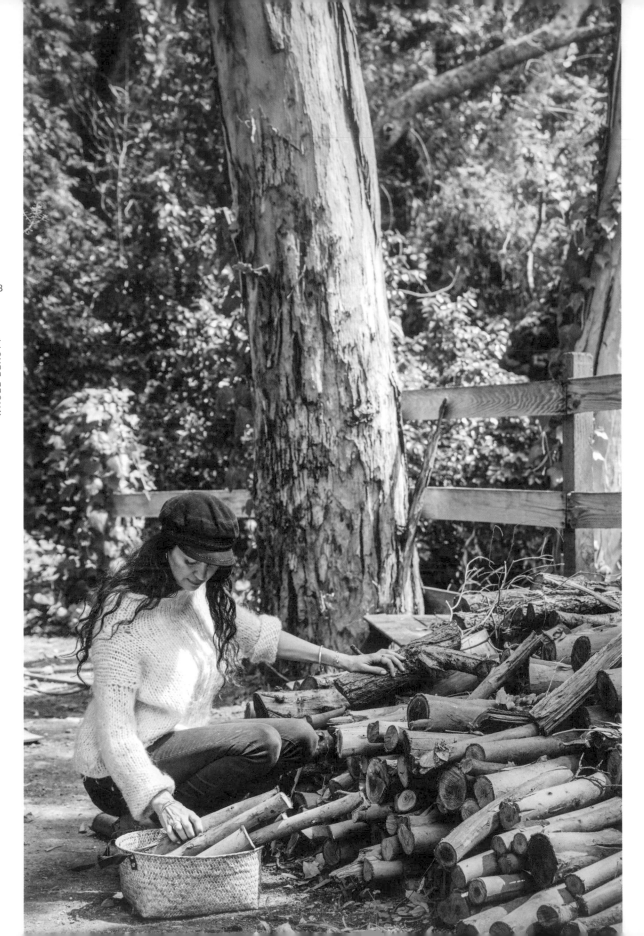

Autumn

Autumn is a time for hearth and home and preparation, for hunkering down and getting ready to nest. Look forward to gathering wood for winter fires and planting bulbs that will bloom in the spring. With the holidays on the horizon, autumn is a time for gatherings. Sage your space (see page 32) and host circles, inviting people into your home to share energy and create warmth. Autumn is also the ideal time to journal, both to reflect on the year that has passed and to anticipate the one to come. A great way to begin the journaling practice is by setting aside a few minutes first thing in the morning or before you go to bed at night to write whatever comes into your head. Start with as little as five minutes, and don't judge or edit the words as they flow from your hand onto the page. Just write. Increase the time if you have a desire to continue writing.

Winter

Winter is a time to nourish yourself and regain your strength. There is something so beautiful about living in sync with nature, and in winter you can be as quiet as the snow-covered ground. Hibernate. Eat root vegetables to ground yourself to the earth, make soups to nourish yourself and those you care about, and light candles to bring warmth into your home. If you are the type to bundle up and go for walks outdoors, you can look for treasures and make winter mandalas with pinecones, evergreen branches, and winter berries.

Phases of the Moon

Birth, life, death, and renewal are all reflected in the cycle of the moon, and menstrual cycles often mirror the moon's cycle.

The new moon is a time for starting projects and increasing abundance. The full moon is a time for healing rituals, finishing projects, and gathering the moon's energy. The waning moon is a time for clearing and cleansing. I like to do an intention-setting ritual with the new moon, writing down my intentions on a piece of paper, then waiting until a full moon to throw the paper into a fire to release them.

Timing your beauty rituals to coincide with the phases of different moons can be a powerful way to reconnect with nature and the cycles within your life. I like to use scrubs on the new moon, then replenish with nourishing masks on the full moon.

Native Americans had different names for each full moon, and the names often varied depending on tribe and region. Consider adding a moon calendar to your sacred space (there are several beautiful, artisan-designed ones available), and let these names guide what you add to your altar throughout the year.

NATIVE AMERICAN
MOON GUIDE

JANUARY
Wolf Moon

FEBRUARY
Snow Moon

MARCH
Worm Moon

APRIL
Pink Moon

MAY
Flower Moon

JUNE
Strawberry Moon

JULY
Thunder Moon

AUGUST
Sturgeon Moon

SEPTEMBER
Corn Moon

OCTOBER
Hunter's Moon

NOVEMBER
Frost Moon

DECEMBER
Long Nights Moon

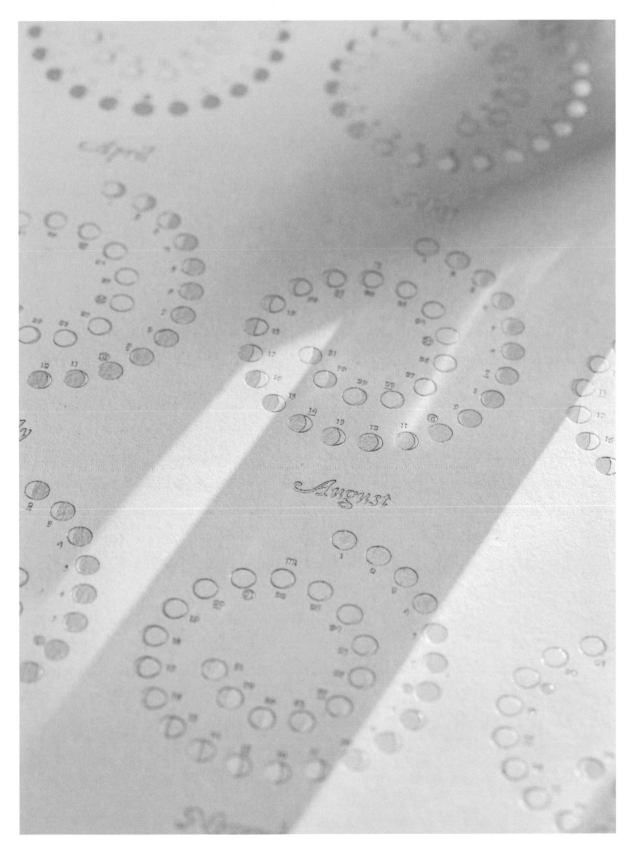

Crystals

People who are into crystals often say that you don't own crystals, you simply take care of them for a while, and they come and go as they please. I certainly believe this, though sometimes it is heartbreaking! I had a beautiful collection of crystals that I had found (or that had found me!) on Mount Shasta—they were tiny little gems of watermelon tourmaline and rose quartz, and from the moment I saw them, I knew they were magical.

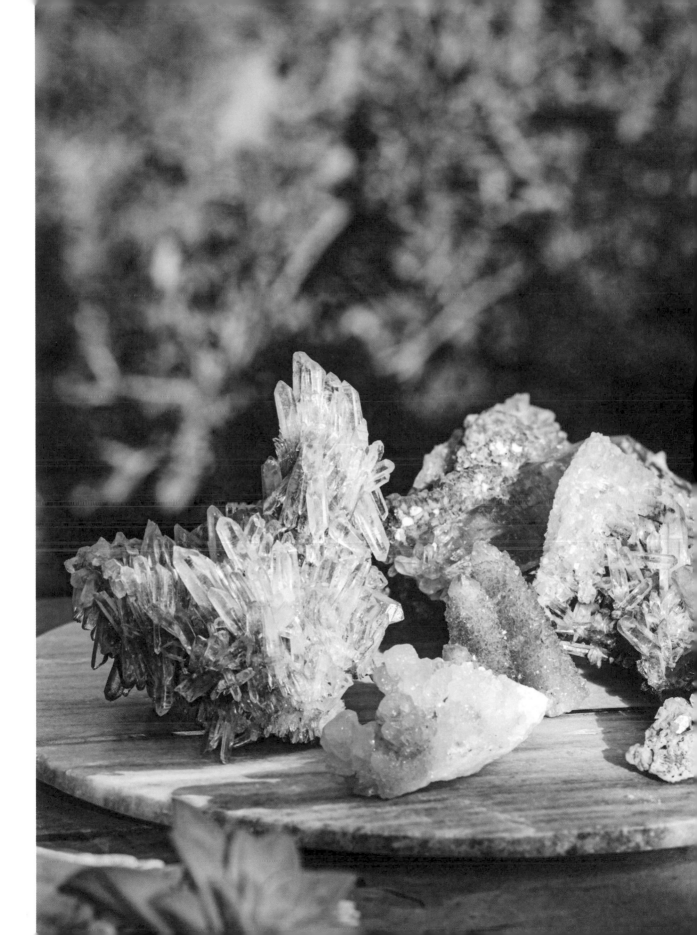

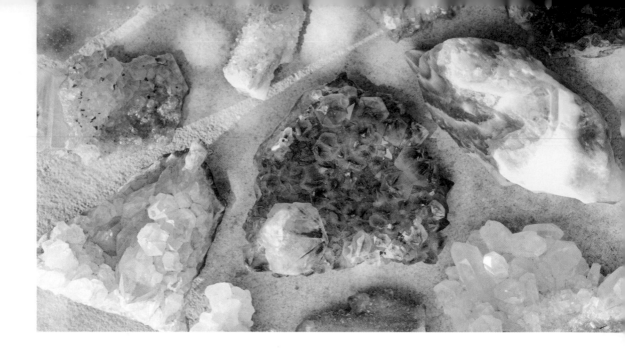

One New Year's Eve, I went to a friend's party in Malibu, and because I was feeling vulnerable that evening, I took my crystals with me. Somehow I lost them. I was devastated and looked for them up and down the street, even to the dismay of my friend, who thought I was overreacting.

"Shiva," another friend said, "maybe they just walked away because they were done." Even if that was true, it was hard to hear. I still miss them to this day!

Aside from just their sheer beauty, crystals help us bring the desired energy and vibrations into our lives. I like to meditate on a crystal's distinct qualities, and I also use them on my altars to draw in goddess energy. I lay them on myself during body work and add them to baths for clearing, balancing, and healing. I also carry them with me—like on that fateful New Year's Eve— for extra grounding and support during hard times.

Shopping for crystals is like falling in love. You are drawn to certain crystals for specific reasons, so go with your gut and don't overthink it! It's important to note that the color varies from crystal to crystal, and just because you might come across a crystal that does not match its typical color, it doesn't mean that it's less powerful.

MY FAVORITE CRYSTALS

Amethyst

A lovely lavender, amethyst helps to heal the heart and soothes the nervous system. It is the stone of spirituality and contentment, and it promotes calm.

Black Tourmaline

Dark and shiny, black tourmaline releases negative energy, provides protection, and shields from harmful EMF rays. I keep a large piece of black tourmaline by my computer.

Citrine

A honey-yellow hue, citrine promotes abundance and financial stability. A stone of manifestation, it can help bring your desires into being.

Jade

A delicate mint green, jade balances energy and can help bring in prosperity. It calms the mind and enhances our life force. Jade has been said to bless whatever it touches.

Labradorite

A range of different, subtle colors, labradorite inspires intuition and aids in connecting to higher realms and overcoming emotional blocks.

Moonstone

Shimmery like a pearl, moonstone connects us to the feminine by representing the power of the moon. It can also help to enhance our intuition, balance the chakras, and promote a sense of calm.

Morganite

A pale-pink, peachy stone, morganite is a mysterious crystal. It helps to heal and release old wounds and traumas, and it is used to bring in your soul mate.

Rose Quartz

A lovely light pink, rose quartz has a soft, feminine energy that inspires beauty. It helps with healing, to open the heart, and to bring love into your life.

Smoky Quartz

A clear gray, smoky quartz helps with organization and clarity. It releases negativity and promotes protection. It is a powerful grounding stone that is often used in meditation. It is helpful in praying to ancestors and anchoring yourself in the natural world.

Tiger's Eye

A beautiful blend of dark and light brown, tiger's eye inspires and aids in decision making. It releases negativity and provides clarity. It was often used to create the eyes in statues of Egyptian deities because it was thought that with tiger's eye, they became all seeing.

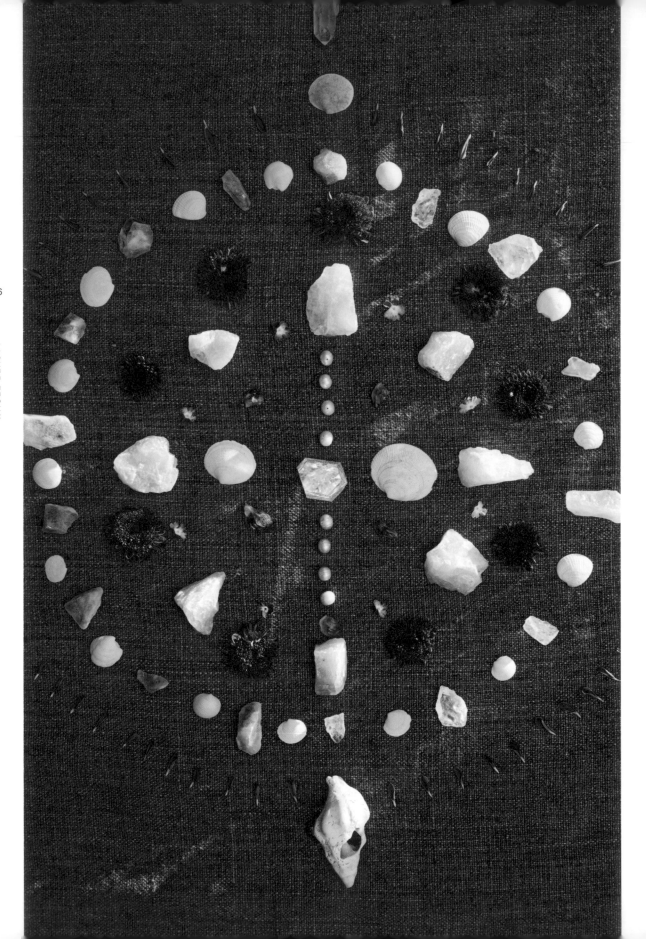

Charging Crystals

To charge a crystal is to imbue it with energy and intentions. There is no right or wrong way to charge crystals. You can charge your crystals anywhere you think they will absorb positive energy. I like to bathe them in sunlight or moonlight (I tend to see sunlight as a more masculine, active energy and moonlight as a more feminine, receptive energy). I also like to take them to Kundalini classes. You can charge your crystals on your altar too. Simply place the crystal on the altar, light a candle, and spend a few moments meditating, imagining your intentions and energy going into the crystal.

Cleansing Crystals

Cleansing crystals allows them to release all of the energy that they have absorbed. Always cleanse crystals before their first use, and cleanse them after rituals or experiencing tough situations. Charging crystals under the sun or moon also clears them, but once a month, fill a big bowl with water, then add a handful of pink Himalayan salt, place your crystals in the saltwater, and let them sit overnight. In the morning, dispose of the water by throwing it outside, and rinse and dry your crystals.

Daily Rituals

Morning

Many Eastern philosophies believe that the best time to work on yourself is between 4:00 a.m. and 7:00 a.m. I get up early, often before dawn, so that I can have some time to center myself and prepare for the day before my daughters wake up. I try to start every day with the following practices, and I alter them depending on how much time I have and if I am traveling.

- Give thanks to the sun as soon as I open my eyes. The sun gives light so that we may live, and it is a beautiful thing to greet it every day as it streams in the windows.
- Wake up my face by spraying it with a rose water hydrosol (see page 265), then get out of bed.
- Massage my face with a fragrant, nourishing oil (see page 205), using upward motions, massaging around the eyes and pressing pressure points to relieve puffiness.
- Scrape my tongue (see page 114).
- Do oil pulling (see page 115; sometimes I do just five minutes, if that's all I have time for).
- Sit for a five- to ten-minute meditation (see page 74). I like to sit and look out at the garden, or sit in a quiet spot in the house and light a candle.
- Follow with three to five minutes of cat-cow pose (see page 96).
- Have a cup of hot water with lemon.

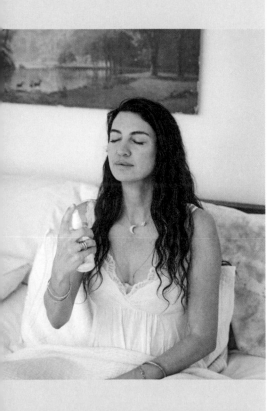

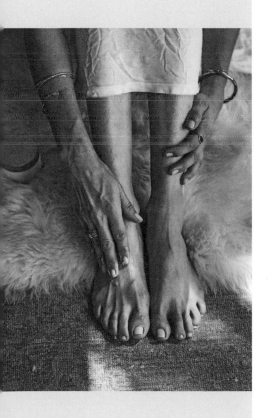

Evening

After I've cooked dinner and I have my house to myself, this is my time to de-stress and release the day. I like to wind down and recharge with the following practices, giving myself time to reflect and practice self-care.

- Light a candle and set some intentions. If I am trying to call in a goddess, I might also add flowers to my altar.
- Put on a recording of a mantra. I like the ones by my Kundalini family, White Sun. These are easily available on Spotify.
- Do dry brushing (see page 116).
- Use a scrub to exfoliate my body and face.
- Steam my face (see page 133).
- Take a bath. I like to add essential oils and/or nourishing ingredients to the water (see page 124). Release all negativity and worry into the bath.
- Get out of the tub and pat myself dry, then anoint myself with oils to moisturize my skin (see page 276).
- Activate my yoni egg (see page 98) and do some meditations.
- Massage my feet with shea butter as a last step before bed (see page 119).

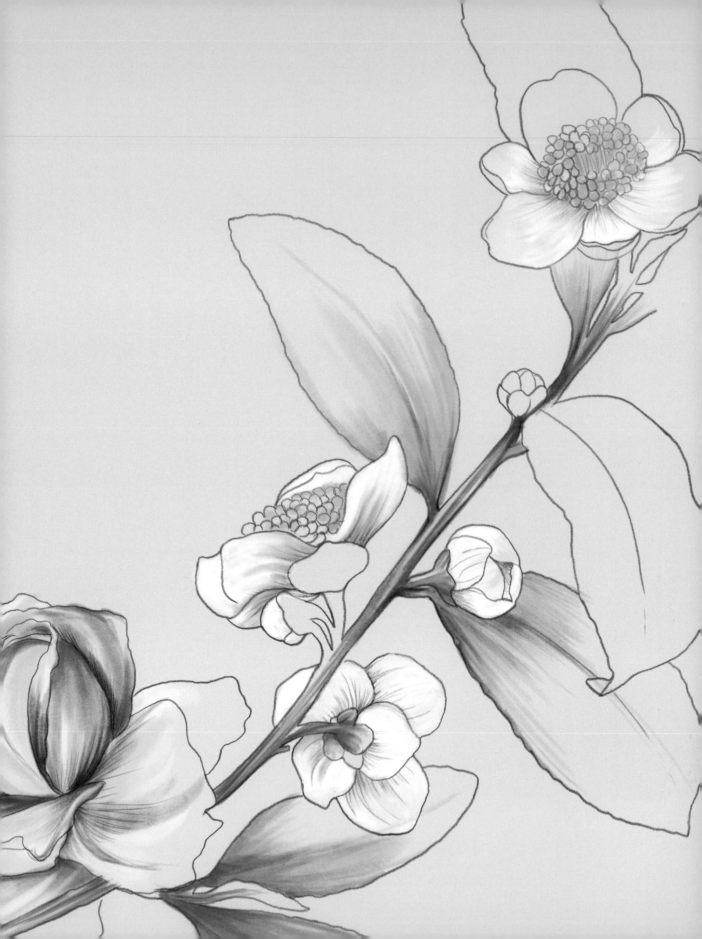

CHAPTER TWO

Kundalini & Mindfulness Practices

I truly believe that there is no outer beauty without inner beauty, and inner beauty starts with a compassionate heart and a mind that is free from fear, worry, and stress—plus we all know stress accelerates aging! Meditation helps to open your heart and calm your mind, but I was always terrified of it because I have such a monkey brain.

I had tried many different forms of meditation, but my brain wouldn't sit still and my thoughts jumped all over the place. I had listened to other people speak about how meditation had transformed their lives, but for me, it created stress rather than alleviated it. Every time I tried, I failed.

When I discovered Kundalini, it was like someone had flipped the meditation switch in my mind and everything was finally illuminated. Through breath, postures, and mantras, Kundalini meditation gave my mind a focus, something to do rather than just sit there, and it got me onto a meditative wavelength.

Kundalini derives its name through its focus on awakening the spiritual energy that is coiled like a snake (a literal translation of the Sanskrit term *kundalini*) at the base of the spine, through regularly practicing meditation, pranayama (breathing techniques), yoga asanas, and chanting mantras. Referred to as "the yoga of awareness" by practitioners, it aims—according

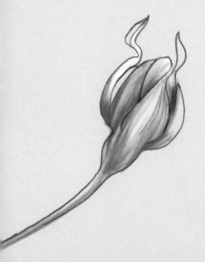

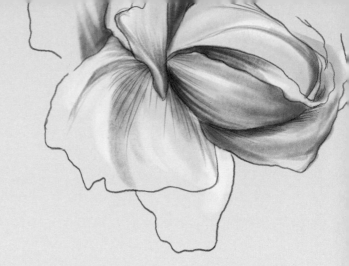

to one of my teachers—"to cultivate the creative spiritual potential of a human to uphold values, speak truth, and focus on the compassion and consciousness needed to serve and heal others."

I first began doing Kundalini yoga when I was pregnant with my older daughter; however, I didn't have a consistent daily practice until I was going through my big life changes years later. After Colette Blu was born, I drifted from the practice, only to return to it with the need to re-create my life after the birth of my second daughter, Charlotte Rumi Rose.

Now, after practicing Kundalini for a few years, I can sit in silence and meditate for twenty minutes or more. When you are engaged in Kundalini, your brain doesn't really have a choice. You have to be present. The reason Kundalini is so effective is because it's physiological. It works on the adrenals, it works on the hormones, it works on the pituitary—it actually works on the entire glandular system.

There are a lot of variations of yoga out there, but I feel that when people come into Kundalini, they really notice a difference, a shift in their life and mind-set.

It is a long-held belief that it takes forty days to change a pattern of behavior. With the first twenty, you're breaking old habits. With the second, you're forming new ones. I always tell people who aren't sure about meditation to try it for forty days and see what happens. The time will pass before you know it, there's no risk of harm, and chances are you will notice profound differences in your life.

Guided Meditations

These visualizations and meditations are an easy introduction to the practice, and the more you do them, the calmer your mind will become and the easier meditating will be. Many people are intimidated by meditation, just like I was, because they think it involves sitting still and in silence for twenty minutes or more. While you will work up to that with some meditations, you can start with these active meditations and do them for just a few minutes or rounds of breath. It really is up to you. Some people may find one minute challenging; others may be able to sit for much longer without feeling anxious.

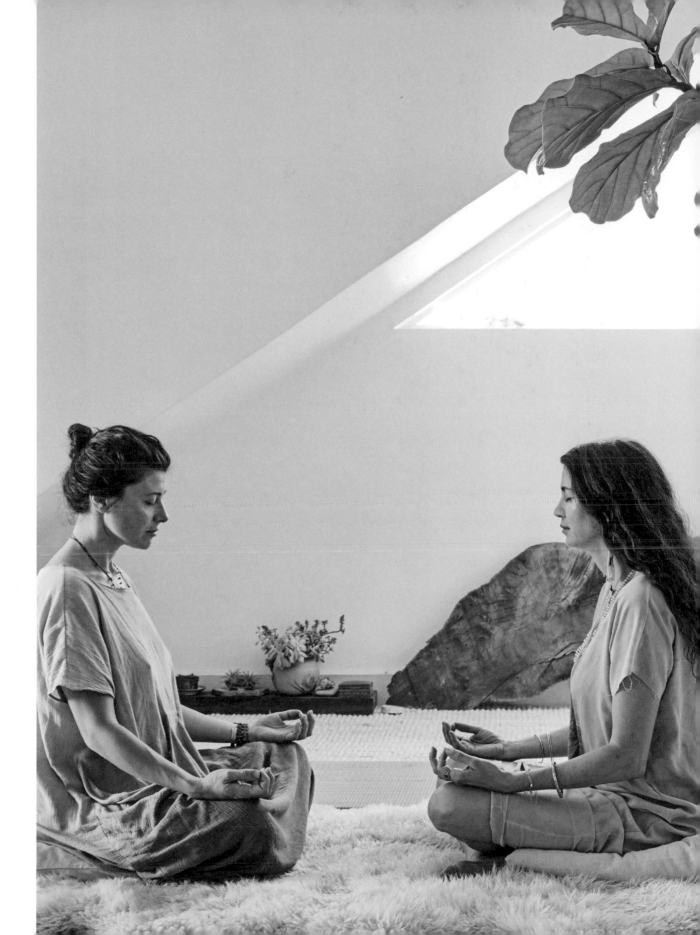

Find a comfortable place to sit or lie, and set a timer. For the duration of that time frame, try to be mindful and keep focus on the meditation. If your mind drifts, don't berate yourself. Just gently return your focus to the meditation and continue. You do not have to do the same meditation every day, though you certainly can, and you can also do different ones in succession.

Guiding Star Meditation

This is great to do when you are dealing with challenges or negative situations and need to be reminded of your powerful inner light and to increase self-love and positivity. As women, we hold a lot of our power in our belly, in our sacrum. Begin by imagining a star there, to increase your positive power, or in your heart, to increase love.

Picture a tiny crystal that is no more than a pinpoint of light. Close your eyes and breathe in and out through your nose.

With each breath, imagine the pinpoint of light growing and getting bigger, until it is a big star right in the middle of your belly or your chest. Imagine all of the rays of the star extending out from you, sharing your beautiful golden light with the world. With every breath, focus on the star. See how it is shiny, bright, sparkly, and white with positivity. It is radiating love.

Imagine each of the star's rays sending that love to the people you care about. I see the rays encompassing my children, my animals, and my home, then my extended family, my work, my friends, and my business. They keep growing, until I send my light to my city, our country, the world, and the entire planet.

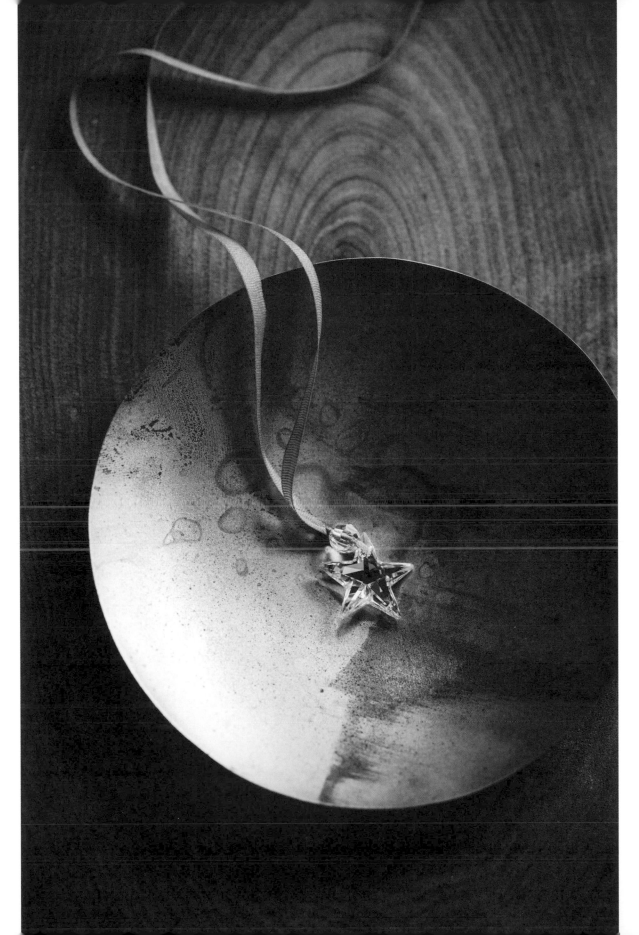

It is a bright golden light that encompasses everything, sending healing love to all corners of our earth. From there, I start to bring it back in. The star gets smaller and smaller with each breath, until it is the size of a silver dollar. Then I let it rest right there, in my chest or my belly, as my power center that lets me carry that healing light and love with me for the rest of my day.

Empowering White Light Meditation

I like to do this kundalini-based meditation first thing in the morning, as it invigorates me and sets me on the course of my day. It floods my body with healing energy, leaving no space for negativity, and illuminates the shadows—think of it as turning on a light to show your children that there is nothing fearsome hiding in the closet. Just as the sun gives the earth the light that allows things to grow, this meditation similarly nourishes mind and body.

Sit comfortably with your arms upstretched in a "V." Close your eyes and breathe normally. Begin by imagining a beam of light coming into your body through your crown chakra at the top of your head. Imagine the light traveling down to your third eye and blessing all of your dreams and visions. (The third eye, which is right where your pituitary gland is, is associated with the god Shiva and has been called the "gateway to the unconscious" because it is the seat of our intuition.)

From there, it progresses into your throat, onto your shoulders, and down your arms. Imagine the white light bathing you all the way to the tips of your fingers.

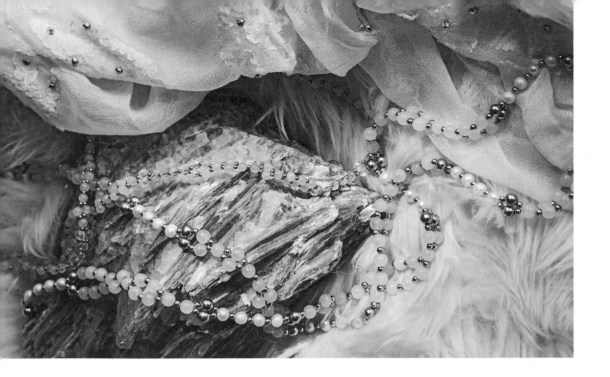

Allow the light to enter and heal your heart, then travel down through your stomach to your root chakra, making you feel grounded and supported. Allow it to travel through your legs, down to your feet and even your toes.

I use this time to remind myself to take it in by just saying "Receive, receive, receive" as the light fills me up.

When you feel that the light has illuminated every part of your body, hold it there for a second, being grateful for how blessed and protected you are in everything you do. Then bring your hands down, outstretched, on either side of your body. As you do so, imagine you're cleansing your aura, sweeping it clean of debris and baggage, negative energy, mental anguish—whatever you're carrying that no longer serves you. Then put your hands on the ground and imagine that you're releasing whatever you don't want anymore into the earth, which is taking it in for you.

This little meditation fills your body with energy and snaps you out of depression or sadness. It is hard to be down after doing this!

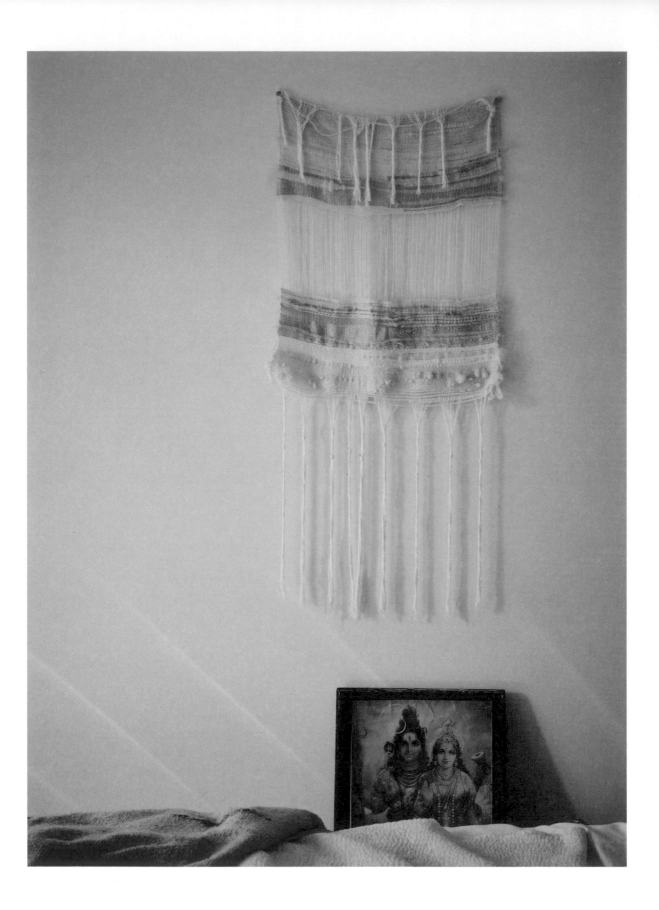

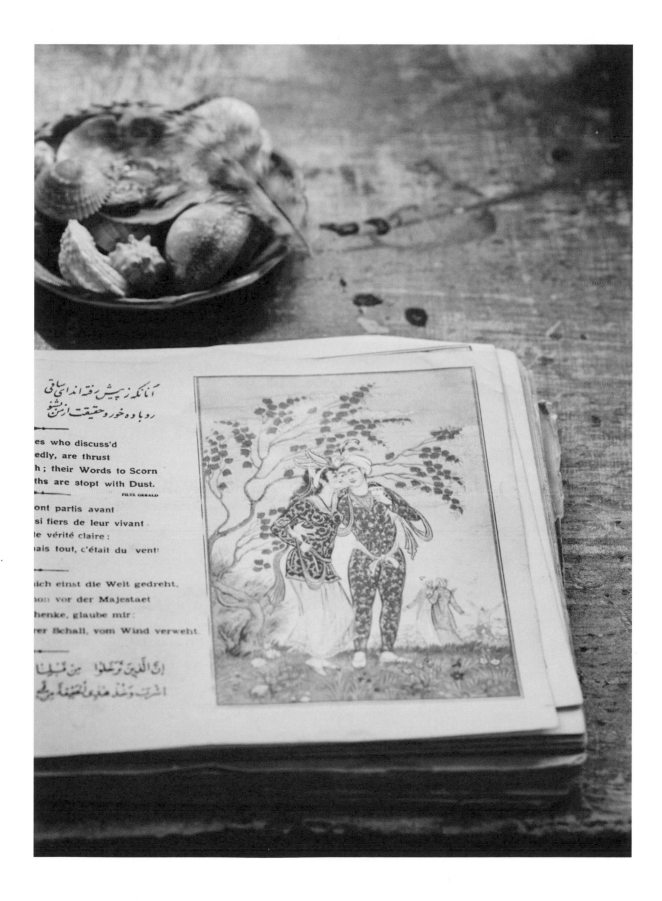

آنانكه زپيش رفته اندای ساقی
روبا ده خور و حقيقت ازين شنو

es who discuss'd
edly, are thrust
h ; their Words to Scorn
ths are stopt with Dust.

FITZ GERALD

ont partis avant
si fiers de leur vivant.
le vérité claire :
ais tout, c'était du vent!

ich einst die Welt gedreht.
on vor der Majestaet
henke, glaube mir :
rer Schall, vom Wind verweht.

إن الذين تخلدوا من قبلنا
اشربت وعند صفر نقيقها برح

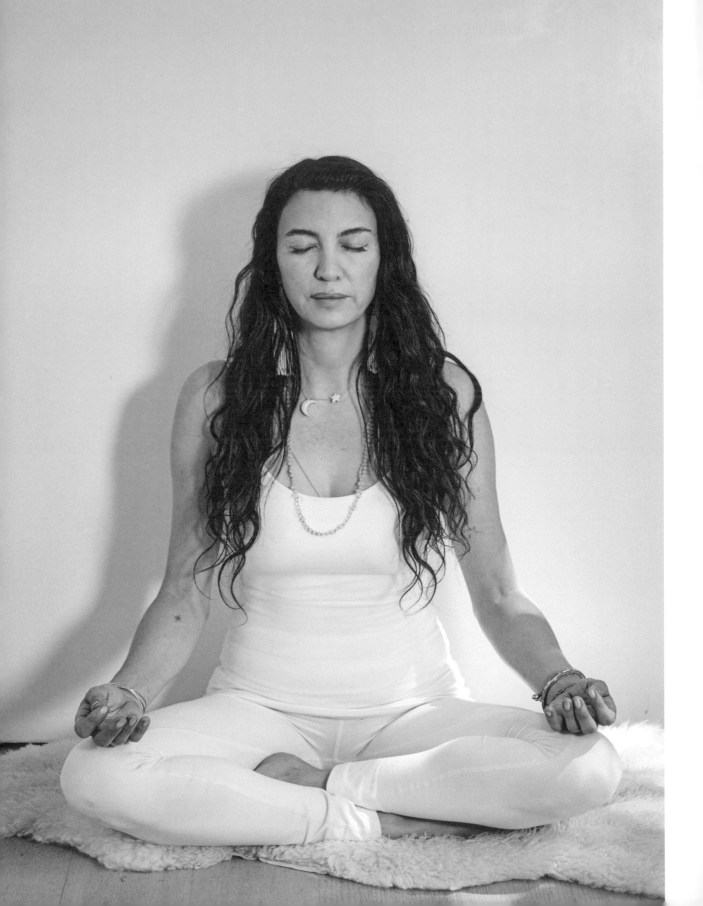

Chakras

Almost fifteen years ago, I was on Kauai and received a body treatment from an angelic woman who told me that my chakras seemed shut down. I was physically, spiritually, and emotionally depleted, struggling to just make it through each day. I was depressed, and my autoimmune issues were flaring up. At the time, I didn't really understand what chakras were, but I knew that something wasn't working, and the words of this woman unlocked a window in my mind.

When I finally started my wellness journey, I found myself returning again and again to my chakras, intent on getting them open and spinning. After years of Kundalini practice, I am well attuned to the powers of the chakras.

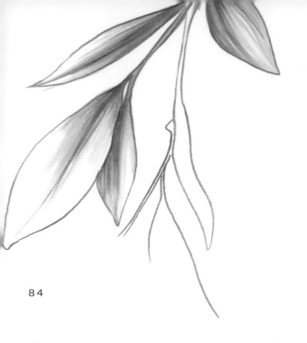

Meditating on certain chakras can help put them into motion, but you can also activate them by massaging the corresponding parts on your body with essential oils (see page 274).

Learning how to recognize and correct imbalances can lead to a greater sense of well-being. Each chakra has a front and a back, the front connecting to your emotions and the back connecting to your will. Each also corresponds to a different part of your physical body. Problems with the chakras in the subtle body, which is the energy field that extends beyond your physical body, will eventually lead to health issues and injury. The chakras' coordinates are represented as a rainbow; red is earth, and the colors get lighter as you move up into the atmosphere. There are seven chakras.

First Chakra

This chakra, also known as the root chakra, is located just below your stomach in the sacral area around the groin. This chakra is about feeling grounded and connected to the earth. It is the chakra of your most basic needs, what you must have in your life before you can begin to ascend to higher levels. When the first chakra is spinning, you feel safe, confident, and supported.

Associations

Color: Red

Corresponding glands: Ovaries, testes

Symptoms of a stuck first chakra: Feeling
   ungrounded, disconnected

Second Chakra

This is the chakra of creativity. It is located in your lower belly and allows you to create something out of nothing, giving birth to everything from children to artistic projects. When the second chakra is spinning, you feel creative and at ease.

Associations
Color: Orange
Corresponding gland: Pancreas
Symptoms of a stuck second chakra: Feeling trapped

Third Chakra

This is your energy chakra and the source of your personal power. It is what enables you to manifest your desires and is located in the center of your belly. When the third chakra is spinning, you feel energetic and driven, equipped with the will and confidence to go after what you want.

Associations
Color: Yellow
Corresponding glands: Adrenals
Symptoms of a stuck third chakra: Feeling tired, frustrated, insecure

Fourth Chakra

This is your heart chakra. It is the seat of love, forgiveness, trust, and compassion and is located in the center of your chest. When the fourth chakra is spinning, you feel deep love for and connection with those around you. You are able to freely give and receive love in all its many forms.

Associations
Color: Green
Corresponding gland: Thymus
Symptoms of a stuck fourth chakra: Feeling lonely, alienated, unable to forgive or accept forgiveness.

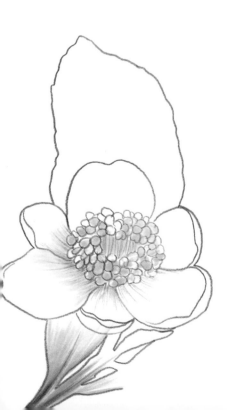

Fifth Chakra

This is the throat chakra and rules your ability to express yourself. It governs communication, speaking, and writing. When this chakra is spinning, you feel that your voice is being heard and that you are empowered to speak your truth and ask for what you want.

Associations
Color: Blue
Corresponding gland: Thyroid
Symptoms of a stuck fifth chakra: Feeling anxious
    about others' opinions of you, unable to speak up

Sixth Chakra

This is the intuition chakra. Located in the center of your forehead, it governs your sixth sense and psychic abilities. The sixth chakra is your inner voice that guides you to trust your instincts. When it is balanced, you are able to tap in to your inner guidance without fear.

Associations
Color: Lavender
Corresponding gland: Pituitary
Symptoms of a stuck sixth chakra: Feeling doubtful,
    indecisive, unsure of what you want

Seventh Chakra

This is the crown chakra. Imagine it as a thousand-petaled lotus flower blooming at the top of your head. When all of your other chakras are spinning, the lotus begins to bloom. You connect to the source of all being and recognize your own divinity.

Associations
Color: Violet
Corresponding gland: Pineal
Symptoms of a stuck seventh chakra: Feeling
    materialistic and not living consciously

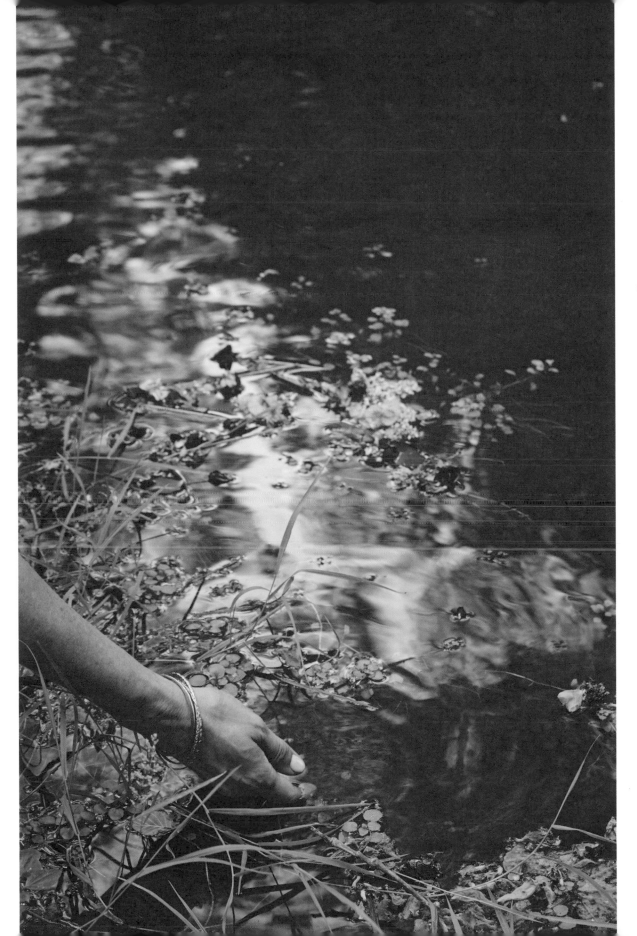

Breathing

Prana, or "breath," is what fuels our life force. Most of us aren't taught how to breathe correctly and usually only do so in a shallow manner. Once you learn to fill your diaphragm and lungs with air, you will notice how much more awake you feel. These yogic breathing methods are also anti-aging because they help awaken the endocrine system and bring more oxygen to the skin and organs.

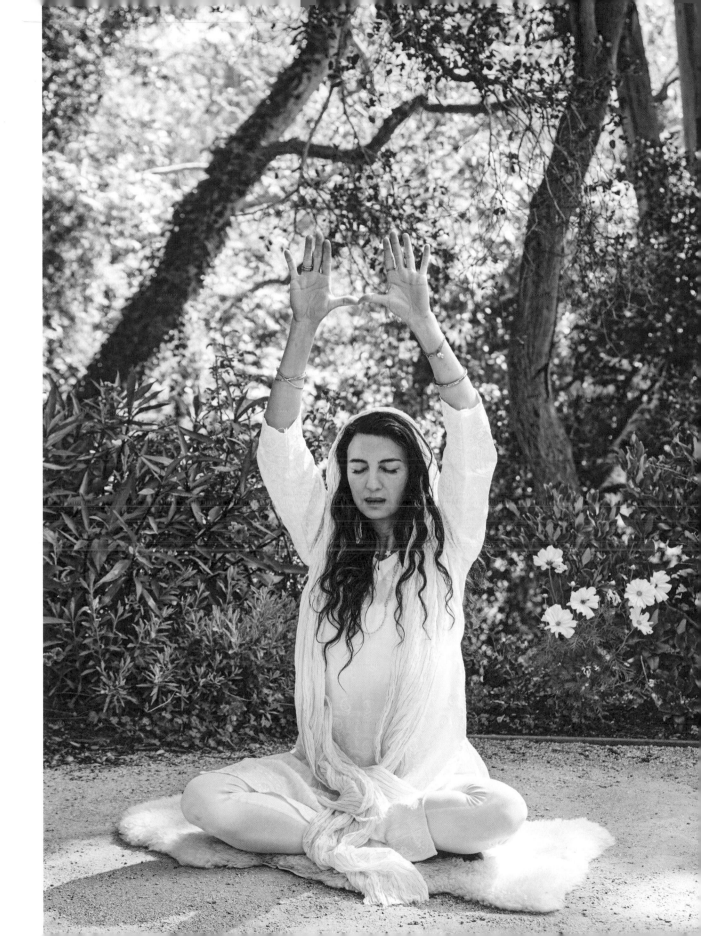

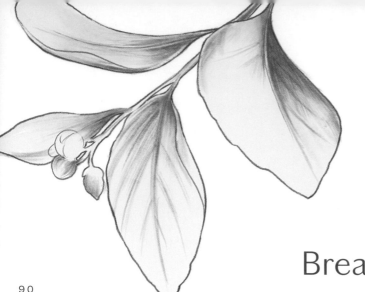

Breath of Fire

In Kundalini yoga, it is said that if you feel down or depressed, it's because you don't have enough prana in your system. Breath of fire, a Kundalini kriya (exercise), remedies this. It is a vehicle for changing your brain chemistry and creating lots of joyful energy. Personally, I notice huge shifts when I utilize breath of fire in my day. It clears my aura and makes it brighter.

For breath of fire, sit in a comfortable position holding your arms up in a "V" above your body. Close the four fingers of each hand against your palms, and have your thumbs out, pointing in toward each other.

Inhale and exhale through your nose, rapidly, and with enough force that you feel your diaphragm moving.

Do this for three minutes. Your arms might start to burn, but they're not going to fall off. After three minutes, bring your thumbs together so that they touch overhead, and uncurl your fingers so that they are pointing up. Tighten up your pelvic floor (almost like you're stopping the flow of urine), which will enable all of the energy you've collected to spiral up your spine toward your head.

This kriya will clean your digestive system and bring new energy and oxygen to your brain and bloodstream, all in just three minutes that will leave you with a new vitality for the rest of your day. Over time, it can change your cells.

Alternate Nostril Breathing

Alternate nostril breathing, or *nadi shodhana*, has powerful beautifying effects. *Nadi* means "energy channel" and *shodhana* means "cleaning" or "purifying." This technique keeps the mind calm and releases tension and fatigue. The alternate breathing cleanses your lungs, which oxygenates the skin, brightens the eyes, opens energy channels, and promotes better sleep. Alternate nostril breathing gets the two sides of the body to work together. The left side is the feminine nurturing, calming side and the right side is the masculine active, competitive side.

First, use your right thumb to close off your right nostril. Then inhale slowly through your left nostril. Pause for a second with your lungs full. Now close your left nostril with the ring finger of your right hand, and take your thumb off your right nostril. Exhale through your right nostril.

Begin the cycle again by inhaling through your right nostril. Pause again when your lungs are full. Use your right thumb to close off your right nostril, release your left nostril, then breathe out through your left nostril. This is one round.

Start slowly with one or two rounds and gradually increase. Never force your breath, especially if you have a stuffy nose or blocked sinuses. Sit quietly for a few moments after you have finished.

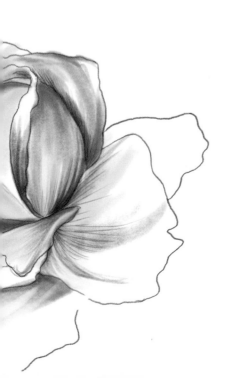

Mantras

Mantras are the sound component of Kundalini, and they are based on the concept of like attracting like. When you speak or chant a mantra, it will help bring the spirit of the mantra into your life. Mantras help rewire the brain so that the neurons fire in pathways that strengthen the body, not deplete it. In short, they help the brain get into a groove more easily, and eventually, that groove becomes automatic. The mantras replace the same negative thought patterns that we repeat over and over, the ones that wear us out and create anxiety.

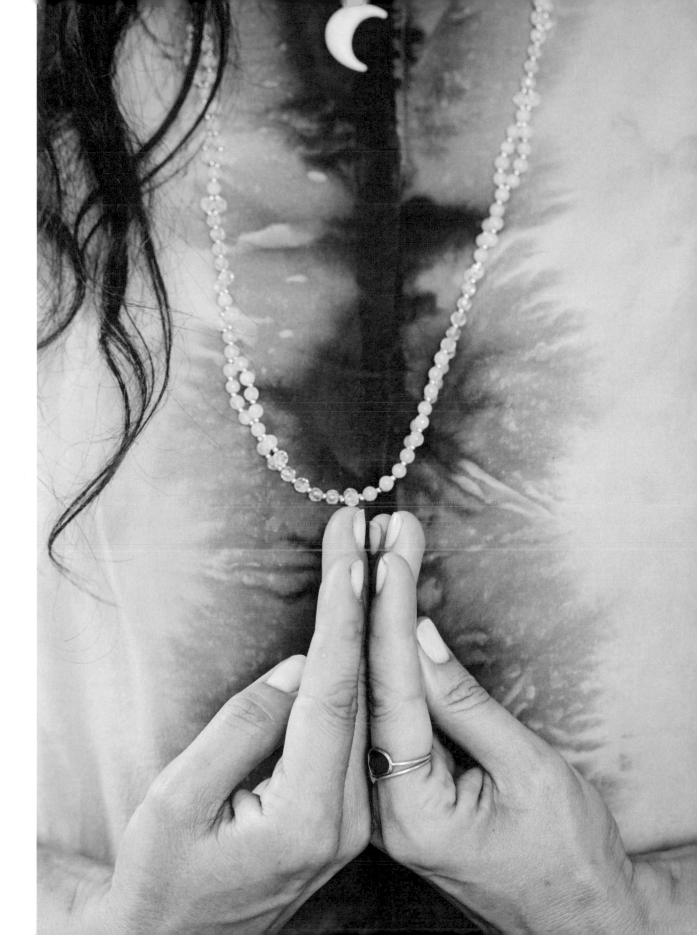

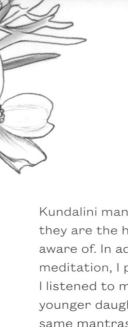

Kundalini mantras are thousands of years old, and they are the highest earthly vibrations that we are aware of. In addition to chanting mantras during meditation, I play them in my house and in my car. I listened to mantras while I was giving birth to my younger daughter, and now she listens to those same mantras when she needs help falling asleep. In Los Angeles, sitting in traffic is a daily annoyance, and several times I've put on a mantra when stuck in a jam and felt my frustration clear right up. Most Kundalini mantras are in Gurmukhi, an ancient Indian language, but some are in English as well (see opposite). The words produce vibrations in different parts of the roof of the mouth, activate chakras and stimulate various areas of the body and brain, and help you to listen to the sound within yourself.

Tuning In

Tuning in is the first step before any chant or kriya. Start by putting your hands together in prayer pose, with your thumbs up against your breastbone. Bringing your hands together is like bringing together sun and moon energy, and marrying the masculine and feminine sides of yourself. Take three deep, cleansing breaths, inhaling through your nose and exhaling through your mouth.

Repeat the Adi mantra, "*Ong Namo Guru Dev Namo*," three to five times. It means "I bow to all that is the divine wisdom within myself," and it connects us to what is known as the "Golden Chain," the lineage of Kundalini masters before us. It also opens our spiritual channel so that we may receive the wisdom of the practice and connect with the source of all being.

MANTRAS IN ENGLISH

"I am bountiful, I am blissful, I am beautiful"

"Happy am I, healthy am I, holy am I"

"May the longtime sun shine upon you,
all love surround you, and the pure light
within you guide your way on"

MANTRAS IN GURMUKHI

"Sat Nam"

"I am the truth." It is a very easy mantra and works
for everyone because its meaning is undeniable.

"Ang Sang Wahe Guru"

This mantra is not translatable, but it is the
mantra of ecstasy. Chanting it elevates the soul.

"Ong So Hung"

This is an empowering mantra that opens the heart and
means "Creator, I am thou!"

"Aad Guray Nameh"

"I bow to the primal wisdom." This mantra is used to
invoke the protective energy of the universe.

Cat-Cow Pose

This easy yoga pose wakes up the pituitary gland, the digestion, and the spirit. The pituitary gland is about the size of a pea and is located at the base of the brain. It acts as a main control center to send messages to the other glands and is called "the seat of the mind" since it connects us to our intuition and artistry. I like to do cat-cow first thing in the morning to set the feeling for the day and connect to the source of all being. It also aids in unblocking channels so that energy can flow freely between the higher and lower chakras. According to Guru Jagat, cat-cow helps to pump cerebrospinal fluid through your spine, stimulating the production of collagen, which is what plumps your skin and keeps it firm.

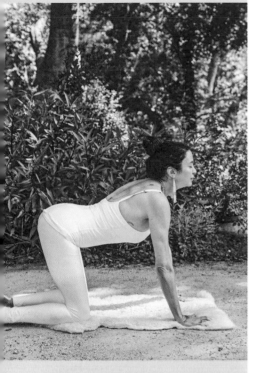

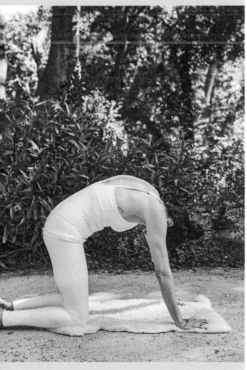

TO DO CAT-COW POSE:

- Come onto the floor on your hands and knees. Make sure your hands are directly under your shoulders, about shoulder-width apart, and that your knees are directly under your hips, about hip-width apart.
- Inhale deeply into cow pose by arching your back to lift your head and chest up toward the sky and allowing your belly and rib cage to expand downward toward the ground.
- As you breathe out, round your spine to draw your head toward your tail, tucking your chin into the chest. Allow yourself to exhale completely, drawing your belly in and up toward your spine as you empty your lungs.
- Move between cow pose and cat pose, filling each movement with a long, full breath (inhaling into cow and exhaling into cat). Start off at a slow pace, then begin to move more fluidly as you feel yourself warming up. Go only as fast as you find comfortable.

Yoni Eggs

Even though my former mother-in-law, Eve Ensler, wrote *The Vagina Monologues*, I was in my forties before I could say the word *yoni* out loud. It wasn't until I started working with the yoni egg, and noticed the correlation between the happiness of my yoni and the happiness of my self, that I felt confident enough to share my use of this practice with others.

Very rarely are women taught to honor their sexuality. Most often, we are taught to alternately fear and protect it, and it becomes a source of anxiety and feelings of inadequacy, not pleasure. But this is an exciting time because women are discovering ancient practices that can help them connect to this inner power.

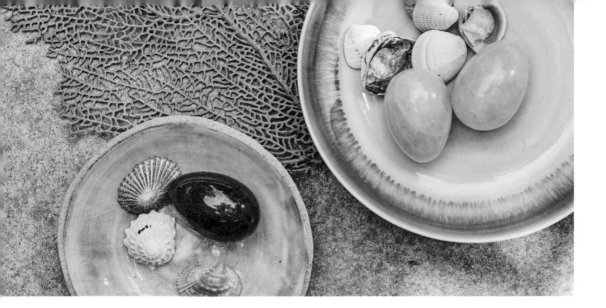

The chakra associated with the yoni is connected to our will, power, and discipline, so if these areas aren't toned, we can see the effects in other areas of our life. Lately, the tradition of using yoni eggs has helped me reconnect to my higher self, pay tribute to the divine feminine, and tune in to joy. The practice of yoni eggs has increased pleasure in all areas of my life.

The word *yoni* means "sacred space" and is the symbol of the goddess, or Shakti, in Hinduism. The practice of yoni eggs was started by the empresses and concubines of ancient China. The yoni practice has so many benefits: strengthening the pelvic floor, maintaining healthy reproductive organs, and enhancing sexuality and receptiveness. It can help balance hormones, and it prevents the decline of nerves in the bladder and uterus.

The yoni is where many women connect with their intuition, their power, and their wisdom. It is this inner sanctum that we can access when it is not in use creating life. More than 50 percent of women in the United States have a problem with incontinence or having orgasms. Because these subjects are not often discussed, there is some controversy surrounding the yoni egg practice, which is to be expected when dealing with an intimate topic. There is plenty of information out there, and differing views on the subject, so I feel that every woman can do her research and listen to

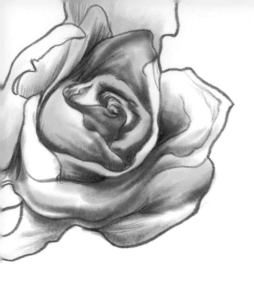

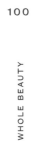

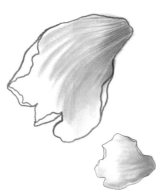

her own intuition when deciding if the practice is for her. Sadly, you rarely hear the kind of outrage that has been directed at yoni eggs directed at other things women place in their yonis, such as dildos made with phthalates, BPA, and toxic plastics or tampons made with pesticide-laced inorganic cotton. To me, those things are way more frightening than a beautiful yoni egg. The important issue, though, is to make sure you learn from a certified expert, like Saida Désilets or Layla Martin, and purchase *only* real gem yoni eggs (both Saida and Layla sell them through their websites; see Resources). You are placing this gem inside your sacred space, so you want to ensure that it contains all the powerful elements of the precious stones and nothing fake. You also need to make sure it is cared for and kept clean. Traditionally, yoni eggs are made from nephrite jade, which is why they're often referred to as jade eggs. I prefer jade, and many experts recommend it, but some women also use rose quartz or black obsidian.

Don't get frustrated if you don't feel anything happen right away. It takes around a month of daily use to really start perceiving the results. Now, of course, I miss this practice if I don't do it; I've become much more sensitive. I have also seen a difference in my cycle. I had hormonal imbalances, and the yoni egg practice has made my whole cycle much more regular.

It is important to respect the power and sacredness of this space and practice, and I feel honored to be at the forefront of a movement that encourages women to be empowered through self-love, not through surgical enhancements or the latest designer clothes.

Creating a Ritual
Around Your Yoni Egg

First, cleanse and clear your egg. Boil it for five minutes in filtered water. Dry it off and burn some sage around it. Imagine the sage clearing any negative feelings you might have about your sexuality or yourself. Visualize golden light filling the egg with positivity.

In front of your altar, or in another quiet, private space, place the egg before you on a beautiful scarf or piece of fabric.

Lie down on your back and place the egg on your heart, then on your belly. Imagine all of your intentions flowing into the egg. Connect with it, honor it, and give thanks for the healing it will bring you.

Follow with the exercises you have gotten from books or an expert. Specific instructions come with each egg, explaining exactly how to insert it. Don't get discouraged—remember, it's a practice. It is vital to follow all tightening with release, since the idea of release and expansion is at the heart of the practice.

When you're finished, clean the egg with warm water, wrap it in silk, and store it on an altar. It should take a sacred place in your life.

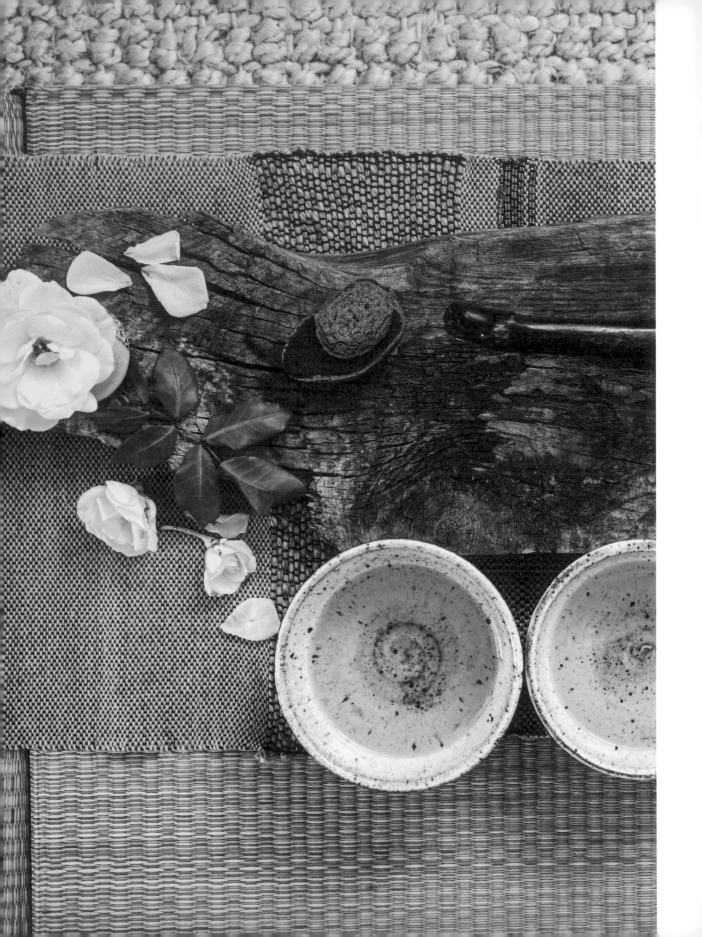

Tea Ceremony

I was introduced to the way of tea—*cha dao*—by my tea sister Tien Wu (Baelyn Elspeth). I had a very visceral reaction the first time I sat in on a tea ceremony. I didn't understand why we were sitting in silence and why we were drinking this tea. I was frustrated and agitated, and I didn't think I would be participating in the tea ceremony again anytime soon.

Because a lot of the sisters in my community practice tea ceremony, I soon found myself sitting in on my second ceremony, and this time my reaction was a complete reversal, as I had pushed through my previous resistance. I started crying, and I found myself deeply moved by the presence and power of tea. Rather than being annoyed by the silence and the stillness, I became aware that this was the very purpose of practicing tea ceremony: to slow down enough that you become one mind that is fully present and in the moment.

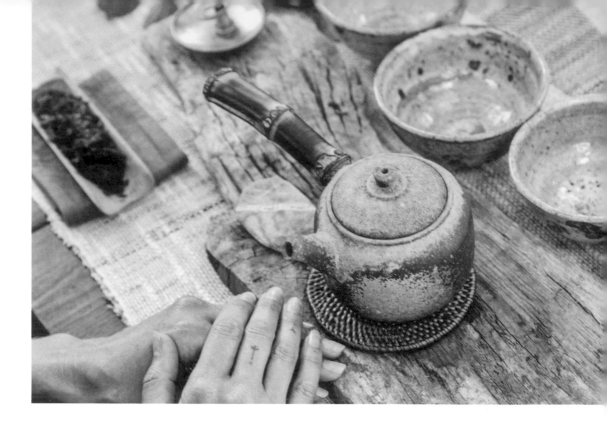

You hear a lot of talk in the media about mindfulness, and the tea ceremony is a mindfulness practice. You have to be totally present as the water boils, as the leaves steep, and as you pour and drink the tea. As I began to appreciate and understand the tea ceremony, I realized how wonderful it was for me. I have a very active mind, and this ceremony gave me a focus for my meditation. It allowed me to let my feelings pass without judgment and to remain still and calm.

I practice tea ceremony with an organization called Global Tea Hut, and my teacher, Wu De, often talks about the tea ceremony as a way of connecting to nature. Many of us live in fast-paced urban environments and often fail to take notice of the natural world around us. The tea ceremony allows us to slow down enough to connect with the spirit of the earth. When I went to China to learn more about tea, the group that I traveled with worked on organic farms, harvested leaves, processed them over fires, and even visited the studio of a master potter who makes beautiful clay vessels that we drank from. This trip deepened my love and appreciation for the process of preparing tea for ceremony, because I got to experience firsthand how labor intensive producing it really is. We could pick leaves for a full day and still barely have what we needed for a pot of tea.

Wu De taught me a simplified version of the traditional Japanese tea ceremony. Ancient Chinese and Japanese ceremonies celebrate nature by incorporating all of the elements: water, the fire and air used to boil the water, and the earth represented by the tea itself and the clay cups. Sometimes we will also burn incense during the ceremony to represent ether. We often practice outside, and a few years ago, I commissioned a craftsman from Ojai to build a small teahouse in my backyard, which has become my refuge. I drop into a deeper place when I am listening to the birds and feeling the breeze purifying me. I always see butterflies fluttering by and hear frogs singing. Drinking tea in my teahouse feels like entering into a whole new realm. Tea is a medicine, and it brings people together. It makes it possible to sit down with a stranger, share a cup, and develop a connection without saying a word.

Starting your own tea practice is very simple, and you don't need much equipment. Begin with organic tea from a reliable source such as Global Tea Hut or Living Tea (see Resources) and clay cups/bowls that are nontoxic and pleasing to you. My favorite cup was given to me by Tien Wu. It was a gift when I first started practicing, and it means a lot to me.

It took me years of being the water bearer for Tien Wu before I felt confident enough to serve tea. Although the practice is very simple and made for anyone to do, it also requires specifics that come from putting in the hours to learn and absorb all of the details.

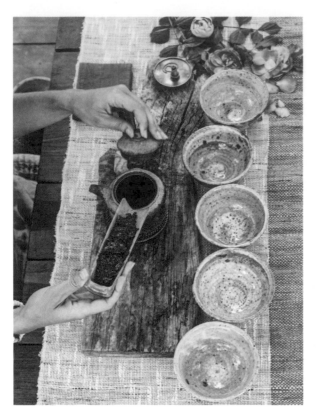
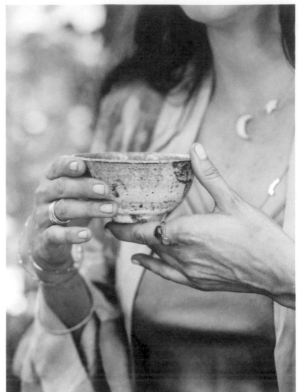

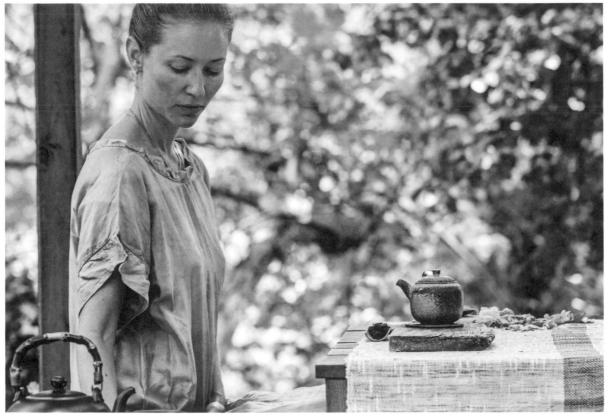

Practicing Tea Ceremony

- Organic tea
- A teakettle
- A nontoxic clay teapot
- Nontoxic clay teacups (Global Tea Hut sells beautiful cups and teapots that are handmade by artisans in China; see Resources)
- Spring water
- Incense
- An offering (like a flower in a vase) that helps to decorate the space for the ceremony

TO PREPARE THE TEA:

Heat the water in a traditional teakettle until it is just about to boil, then transfer it to the teapot that you will use for the ceremony.

Put a few tea leaves in each cup/bowl, and watch them unfurl when you pour in the hot water. As with every practice, preparing tea becomes a ritual when you bring in mindfulness and intention. As the tea blossoms, really take in the history of what you are drinking. Sit outside if you can, and empty your mind of everything else by paying attention to what is around you: the sounds of nature, the feel of the warm cup in your hand, and the taste of the tea on your tongue. Sip in silence. When you are done, make an offering to tea and the earth by tossing your leaves on the ground, rather than in the trash.

KUNDALINI & MINDFULNESS PRACTICES

Falling into the Wells of Tea

A STORY ABOUT MY TEA TRAVELS

Surrounded by cypress trees, wild mint bushes, and rose gardens, the roads were dusty and meandered among abandoned buildings. One had to be alert because of the random wells that littered the earth. "Stay away from the wells, Shiva! You could fall in and be lost forever." Being a curious and rebellious spirit, I would dismiss my mother's warnings and find myself near the deserted wells, peering in, in search of fairy worlds, lost kittens, and a way to fill up my lonely child heart. This memory of the beautiful villages of Iran, this memory that is linked to who I am at my core, comes flooding in as I peer into an abandoned well in a Chinese village in the lush, green province of Huangshan. I am kneeling to see the bottom of a well, but now my heart isn't a lonely hole wanting to be filled up; now it's rather full from the teachings and healing beauty of tea.

Leaving my younger child, animals, home, businesses, and life is no easy task. As much as I still have the nomadic gypsy longings to travel in my blood, I find traveling difficult. When I heard about the Global Tea Hut trip, my spirit called out a big *yes.* And when I saw the pictures of the Yellow Mountain range, I just knew I had to find a way to go. I know now that it is tea and its spirit that led me to making the trip possible. Months later, when I was climbing those mountains with our group, my yearning to be there had become a reality. This was an example of how we can manifest anything when we are connected to a mission or a practice. Sitting in meditation with my brothers and sisters on those mountains is a moment I will always be grateful for. Spending time on the tea farms, and later watching master Zhou make a teapot, enriched my love for this practice.

The memories, though, that are etched upon and will forever mark my spirit are the ones of being in the village where we learned how to process tea over charcoal. The time when we all sat as one, as a family, under a grandmother tree after an arduous day of tea picking is what I keep going back to—being united through tea with these souls that came from Russia, the Czech Republic, New Zealand, Australia, Spain, the Netherlands, Germany, and Taiwan. Wu De graciously shepherded us, brought us all under his wing, beneath the canopy of that ancient tree so that we could feel tea in its truest form.

Tea has linked me to the earth again, and to a community of like-minded spirits. Tea has reconnected me to my lost childhood by awakening me to the similarities between villages in Iran and in China, as well as those villages we forge and steep through tea. The emptiness I have felt as a result of a tumultuous childhood and broken family is somehow filled with every cup of tea leaves.

Tea ceremony has shown me that self-love and a deep, intimate connection to the source of all being are the only ways we can fill up the empty wells of our hearts. When I knelt down to peer deep into a well on the outskirts of a village in China, it was not unlike peering into my teacup as it's being filled. I don't see an empty well or an empty cup; I see only the capacity for more expansion, more growth, more bonds, more mountains to climb, more tea, more love. . . .

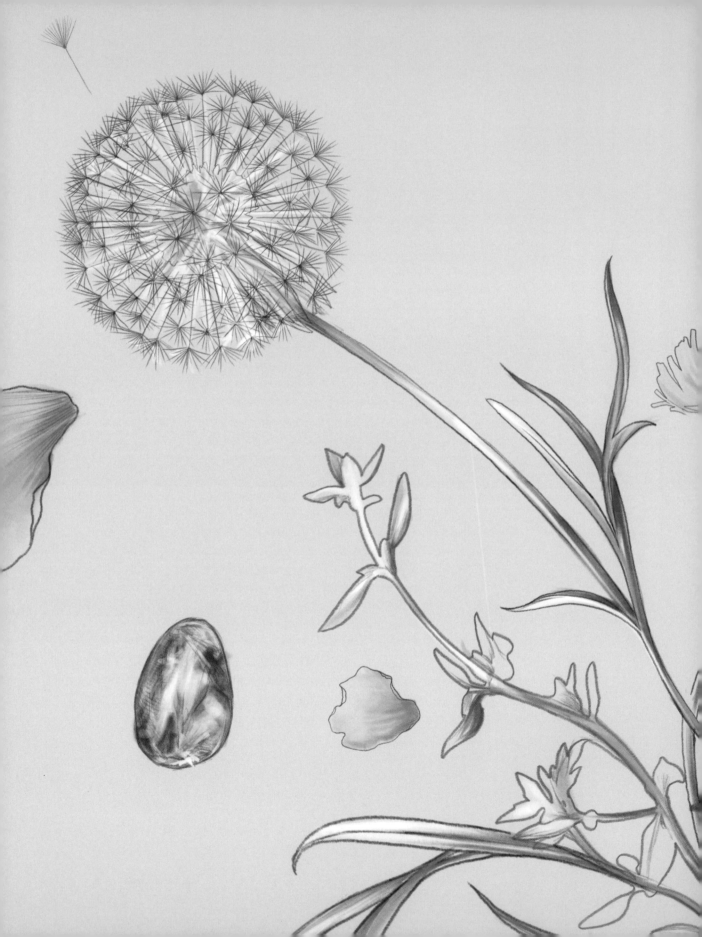

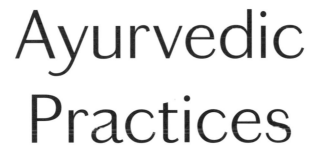

Ayurvedic Practices

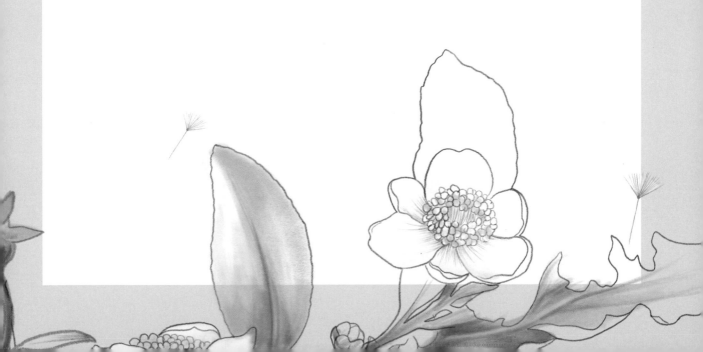

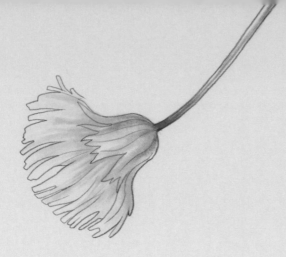

112 A science of self-healing, Ayurveda encompasses diet, meditation, breathing techniques, medicinal herbs, beauty practices, and rituals to heal the body, mind, and spirit. In Ayurveda, inner and outer beauty are intimately related.

Ayurvedic medicine has a rich history, which was originally passed on through the oral tradition, then later recorded in Sanskrit in the four sacred texts called the Vedas. This ancient practice is all about connecting to ourselves and staying in harmony and balance with the natural world. Ayurvedic practices aren't just about preventing diseases rather than simply curing them; they're also about how to live in a state of vigor and energy. In India, more than 90 percent of the population uses some form of Ayurvedic medicine. While it's becoming much more popular here in the West, it's still considered an alternative medical treatment.

The theory behind this medicine is that all areas of life impact one's health. Here in the Western world, we believe in using targeted tactics—generally, prescription medications—to cure specific ailments. Ayurveda views the body as a whole. Like traditional Chinese medicine, Ayurveda is about the mind, body, and spirit connection.

The aim of Ayurveda is to return the body to its original healthy state; true luminous beauty must be supported by health. At the heart of Ayurveda are *ojas*, our life force, the very essence of our health and well-being. They are our honey, the sap in the tree that is our body. Ojas give us the ability to thrive. When our ojas are strong, our bodies are firm and flexible, our skin is clear and glowing, and our hair is shiny and healthy. Ojas also allow us to overflow with love and compassion.

However, the modern world takes its toll on ojas. Constant stress, processed food, technology, overextension, and too much information deplete ojas and dry them out. When we restore them—with meditation, healthy food, and being in tune with the universe—we become radiant.

Ridding your body of waste and toxins helps ojas to flourish, as detoxing allows the system to be nourished. When your body is clear of toxins, it is able to receive the healthy benefits of nutritious food, face masks, and body oils. Rather than promote a harsh, all-at-once approach to detoxing, Ayurveda employs several small daily or weekly practices to help ensure that your body is always detoxing and efficiently processing waste.

Slowly incorporate these practices into your day. You can begin with something as small as integrating fresh produce into your diet, massaging your feet before bed, or dry brushing your skin in the morning. These additions to your routine will help you to continuously keep your body in a rhythm and in balance. Once you know your body, you can adjust certain practices.

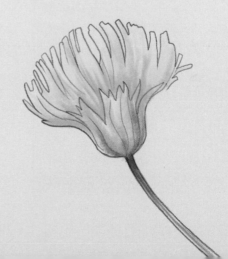

Tongue Scraping

Scraping your tongue every morning can give you clues as to how efficiently your digestive system is functioning. If your tongue is very coated, it usually means there is a lot of *ama*, or toxicity, in your system.

TO SCRAPE THE TONGUE:

- Use a stainless-steel tongue scraper (which you can find online or in most health food stores) or a spoon. Gently scrape from the back or base of the tongue forward until you have scraped the whole surface, which is typically accomplished with anywhere between seven and fourteen strokes. This clears away any bacteria. Scraping stimulates the gastric and digestive enzymes to wake up and start working.
- Rinse out your mouth, and proceed with oil pulling.

Oil Pulling

During the night, as you sleep, your body builds up toxins while it is in the resting, cleansing state. Oil pulling allows these toxins to be released. Oil pulling should be done first thing in the morning, before you have anything to drink or eat. Coconut, sunflower, and sesame oil all work well, but coconut oil has the added benefit of whitening your teeth.

TO PRACTICE OIL PULLING:

- Take a spoonful of oil and swish it in your mouth for fifteen to twenty minutes (this is the recommended period of time, but sometimes I do it for just a few minutes to feel the freshening and teeth-whitening effects of the coconut oil).
- It is important to keep the oil in your mouth and not to swallow it. It also is wise to spit it out in either the toilet or the trash can, as it can clog the sink.
- After you finish pulling, brush your teeth or rinse out your mouth very well.

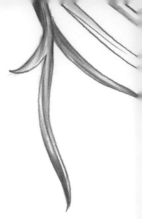

Dry Brushing

The skin is our largest organ and is responsible for 25 percent of the body's ability to detox, yet we tend to focus our beauty routines on the face and hands when the whole body deserves reverence and respect. In addition to being an Ayurvedic practice, skin brushing for the whole body has been used for ages in Scandinavia, Russia, Japan, and Greece and by the Cherokee tribe (using dried corncobs), to name just a few examples. Skin brushing helps rid the body of dead skin and also stimulates the lymphatic and circulatory systems, which assists the kidneys and liver in releasing excess hormones that have built up in the organs.

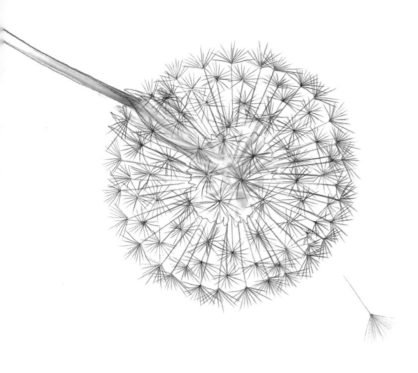

Over time, dry brushing can prevent cellulite and help regenerate collagen, and in the short term, it invigorates and energizes you. As you are shedding dead skin, you are also asking to release what no longer serves you.

Dry brushing should be done before bathing or showering; your skin should be dry.

TO PRACTICE DRY BRUSHING:

- Using a body brush with natural bristles (I like ones that have copper in them to help balance electromagnetic fields), start at the feet and move up toward the torso.
- Using long strokes in the direction of your heart, brush each part of the body six times.
- Brush so it feels slightly painful but good—like when you get a really deep stretch.
- To increase the detoxifying effects, follow with a cold shower.

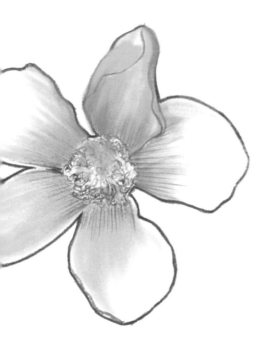

Self-Massage

In the West, we consider a massage to be a special treat, but for many in India, massages are a regular part of life. Babies and toddlers are massaged daily, and when they are a little bit older, they are taught to massage their family members. Women get daily massages for forty days after giving birth. Once you become accustomed to the health and beauty benefits of massages, you won't be able to do without them. Fortunately for our wallets, Ayurveda considers self-massage, or *abhyanga*, to be just as beneficial as a massage given by another.

Set aside some time once a week, or daily if you can, to practice abhyanga, and you will soon see the benefits, including toned, glowing skin; improved circulation; the relief of stiffness in the joints; and the flushing out of toxins in the body. It's also a wonderful way to get to know your own body better.

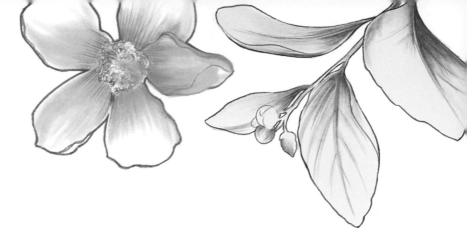

Use sesame, sunflower, or almond oil for massage;
it feels extra luxurious if you warm it beforehand
in a pan of hot water (see page 202).

TO PRACTICE SELF-MASSAGE:

- Apply warm oil generously to your body, beginning
  with your limbs. Use long strokes on your arms and
  legs and circular motions on your joints. Massage
  clockwise to release tension, and include areas like
  your neck and under your arms to target lymph
  nodes.
- Massage your abdomen and chest in broad
  clockwise, circular motions. Follow the path of the
  intestine on your stomach, moving up on the right
  side, then down on the left.
- Apply oil to your crown chakra, working outward in
  circular motions.
- Dip your fingertips in the oil and massage your ears.
- Massage your feet (but make sure to wipe off the oil
  before you walk).
- Throughout the massage, send loving intentions to
  your organs and show gratitude to your body for
  everything it does for you.
- Allow yourself enough time so that the oil soaks
  into your skin before you dress.

If you don't have time for a full massage, you can
always take a small scoop of shea butter and give
yourself a foot massage before bed. This serves
as a form of acupressure, and the shea butter
helps moisturize dry skin. At the same time, you're
honoring your feet—which are your foundation—and
how much they do for you throughout the day.

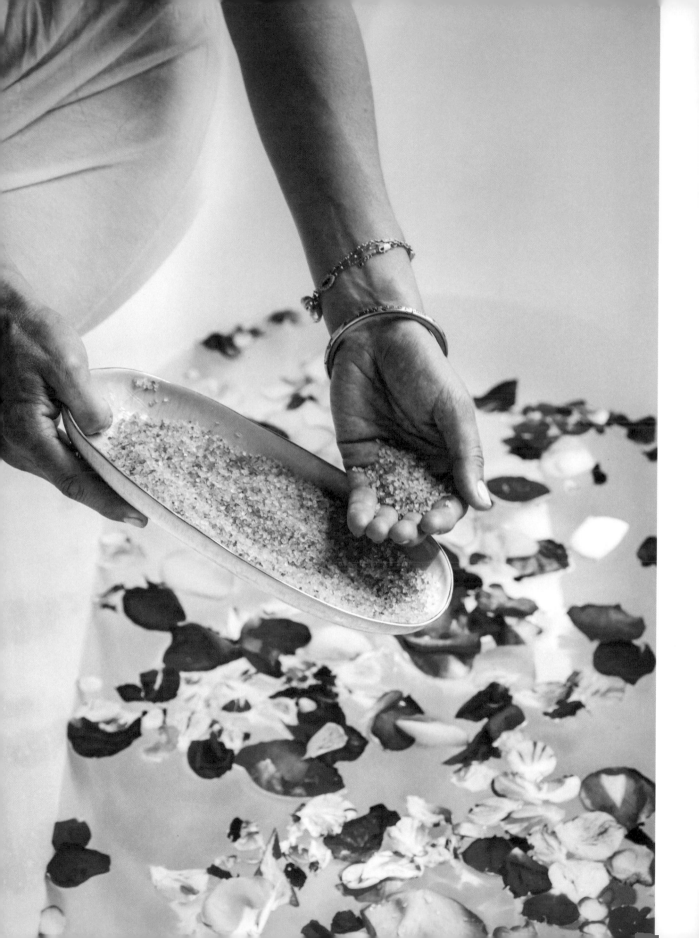

Bathing

In ancient times, bathing was regarded as a gift of health from the gods themselves. Making baths a ritual can be a therapeutic activity. Almost every evening, after I have taken care of my work, my daughter, and my animals, I will indulge in a bath. Taking a bath is the perfect way to have nourishing alone time and create a bit of sanctuary for yourself. Baths are cleansing and can enhance physical and mental energy, remove negativity, and relax your body and mind. They're also a wonderful way to soak up the deeply therapeutic medicine of essential oils and other good-for-the-skin ingredients (see Resources for suggestions on where to shop).

Balancing Bath

122

1 banana, mashed or pureed
1 teaspoon ghee
1 teaspoon plain yogurt
1 teaspoon raw honey
3 tablespoons milk, preferably
 raw (see page 147)

The five foods used in this pre-bath rub are known for balancing the doshas.

Fill the tub with water that is the ideal temperature for you. Mix together the banana, ghee, yogurt, honey, and milk and massage the rub into your skin from your feet to your face. Then soak in the bath for 20 minutes or more.

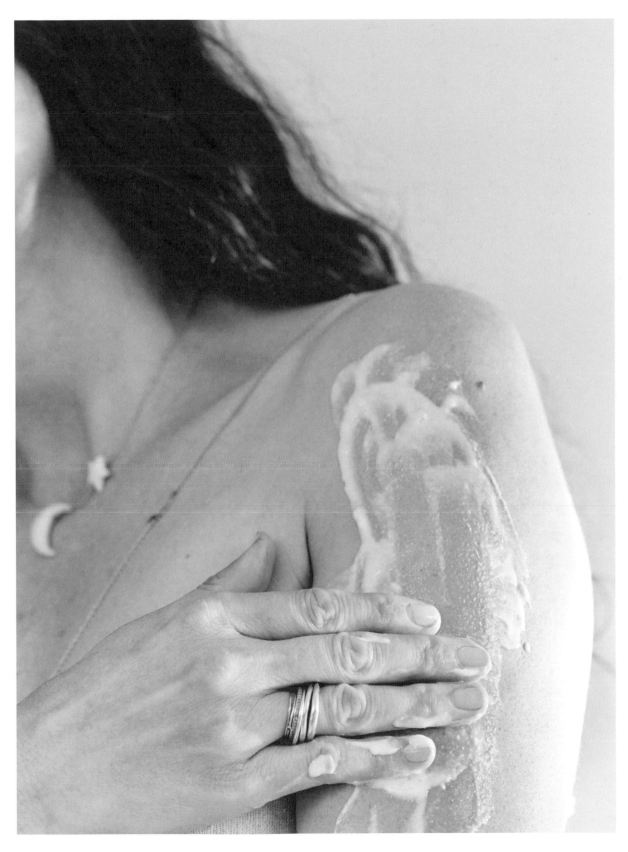

Cleopatra's
Secret Bath Recipe

3 cups cow's or goat's milk,
   preferably raw (see page 147)
1 tablespoon raw honey
10 drops of rose essential oil
A handful of organic fresh or
   dried rose petals

This is an incredibly nourishing treat for the skin. The lactic acid in the milk (I prefer raw, as it has more enzymes and is cleaner) works to remove impurities. The honey is like food for the skin, and rose opens the heart and is anti-aging. After this bath, your skin will be smooth, soft, and opulently scented. This is also ideal for balancing the Pitta and Vata doshas.

Fill the tub with water that is the ideal temperature for you. Add the milk, honey, essential oil, and rose petals before you step in. Soak for 20 minutes or more.

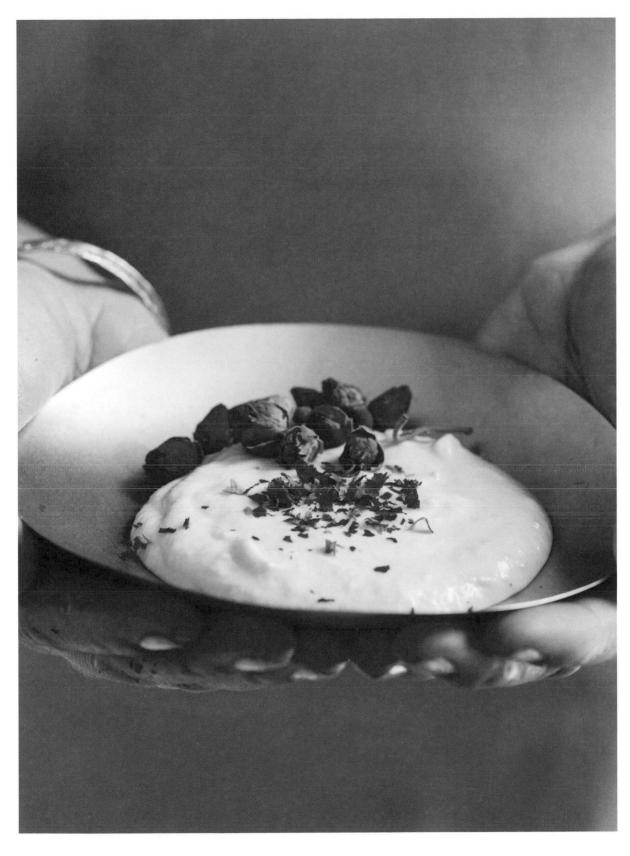

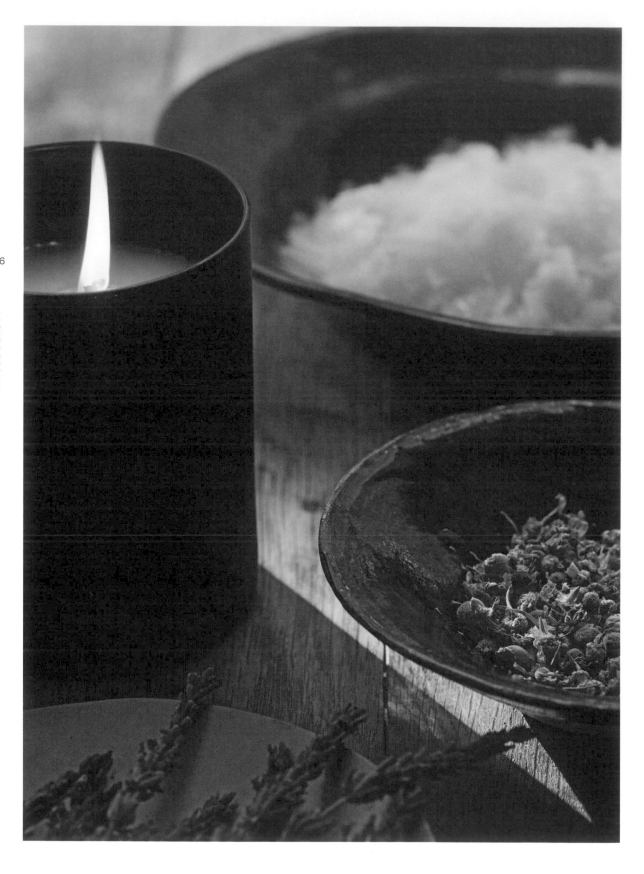

Relaxing
Mineral Bath

1 cup magnesium flakes
10 drops of a relaxing essential oil
  (I like chamomile or lavender)

One of my favorite relaxing baths for all doshas is a magnesium bath. Most of us are lacking magnesium due to depleted foods that are the result of overtaxed soil beds. Magnesium is essential for healthy skin and hair, aids in sleep, and can promote a profound sense of calm and well-being.

Fill the tub with water that is the ideal temperature for you. Add the magnesium and essential oil before you step in. Soak for 20 minutes or more.

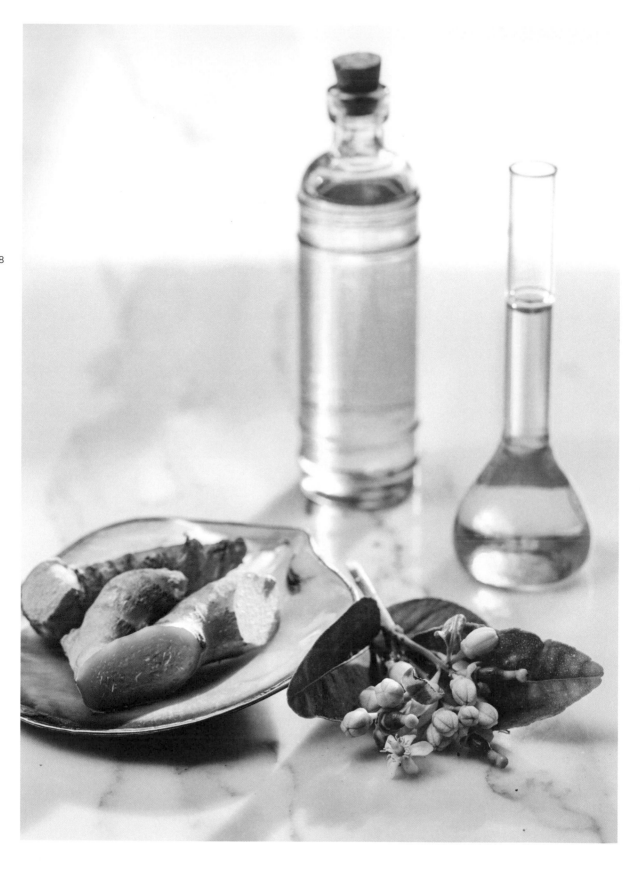

Awakening Bath

½ cup freshly grated ginger, or
   1 teaspoon powdered ginger
1 teaspoon almond oil
10 drops of neroli essential oil

Ginger is an excellent tonic for waking up the senses, and this bath revives and relaxes you before a night out. Or if you are sick with a fever, a ginger bath can help you sweat out toxins and calm sore muscles. It is also good for balancing Kapha dominance.

Fill the tub with water that is the ideal temperature for you. Add the ginger, almond oil, and essential oil before you step in. Soak for 20 minutes or more.

Clearing
Baths

To Bring in Love

A handful of pink Himalayan salt

A handful of rose petals

A handful of dried lavender

Rose quartz crystals

10 drops of rose or lavender
   essential oil

To Cleanse Negative Energy

A handful of sea salt

A handful of white sage

A handful of rosemary

Black tourmaline crystals

10 drops of rosemary or sage
   essential oil

Deborah Hanekamp, a friend and healer, introduced me to the idea of using crystals in a bath, and I have been doing it ever since. When combined with salt, herbs, and flowers in the bath, the crystals' energy is amplified. The use of crystals also makes for a visually beautiful treatment.

Fill the tub with water that is the ideal temperature for you, then add the ingredients of your choosing before you step in. Soak for 20 minutes or more.

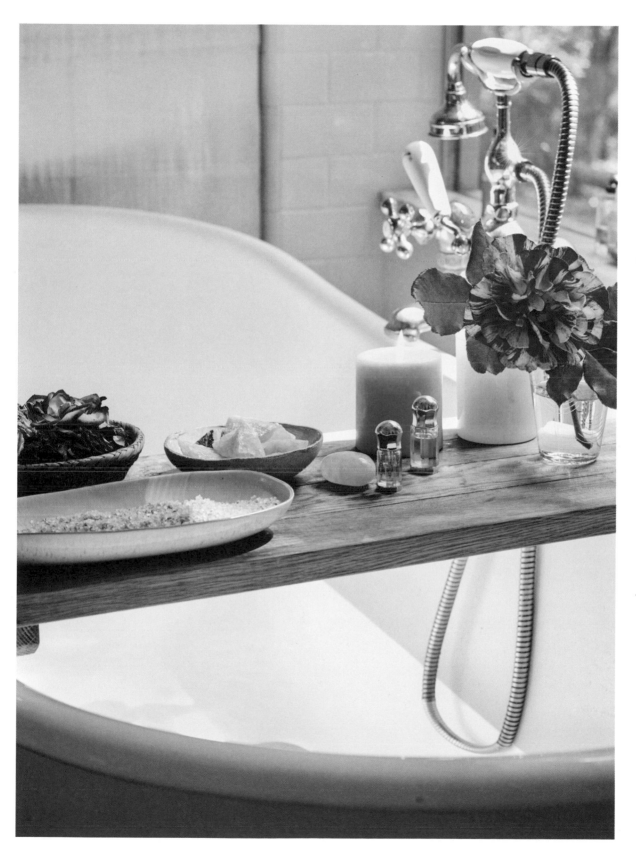

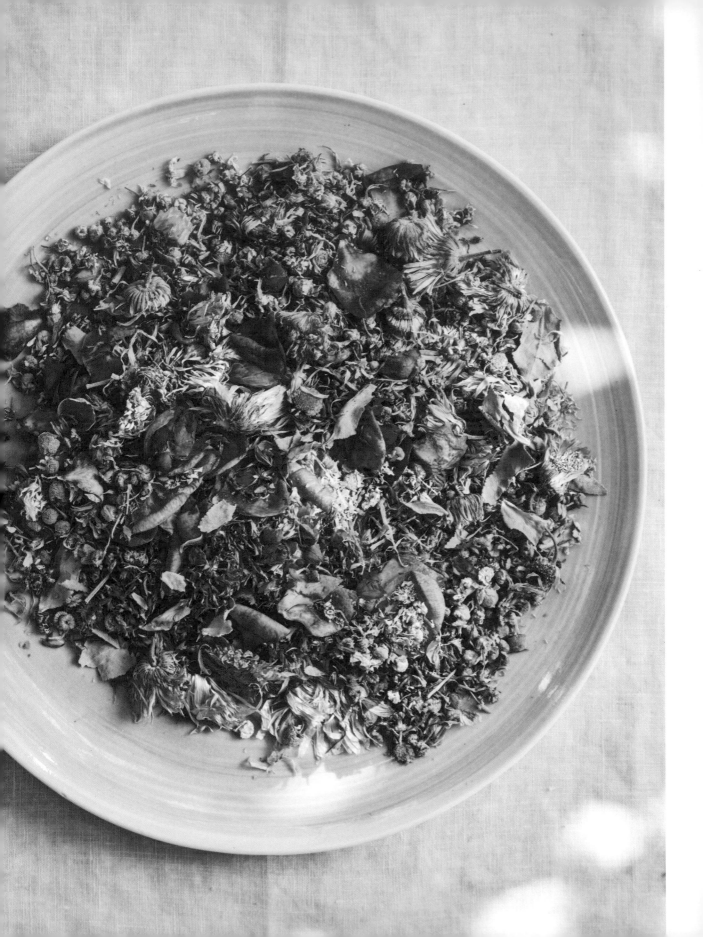

Facial Steaming

Facial steaming is wonderful to do before a bath or shower. It opens your pores, which helps to get rid of impurities and enables your facial products to be absorbed more easily; afterward, you'll be glowing. Steaming also can be a meditative time when you visualize all the incredible properties of the plants nourishing your skin and soul. Make your own custom facial steam by mixing wonderfully fragrant dried herbs with beautiful, colorful flowers. Be sure to look for organic, pesticide-free herbs and flowers from a trusted source.

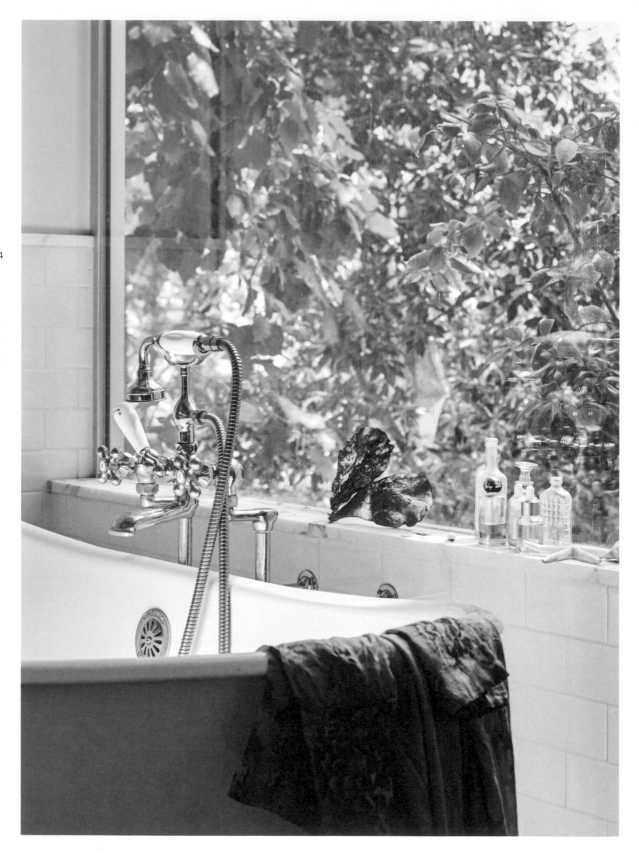

HERBS FOR STEAMING

Calendula
Moisturizes dry skin and has anti-aging properties

Chamomile
Acts as an anti-inflammatory and prevents wrinkles

Cornflower
Soothes and decongests the skin, acts as an astringent, and lightens the complexion

Dandelion
Releases impurities

Raspberry Leaf
Soothes sensitive skin and balances hormones

Rose Petals
Act as an anti-inflammatory and help with sun damage

Sage
Improves circulation

Yarrow
Heals wounds and enhances circulation

ESSENTIAL OILS FOR STEAMING

Bergamot • Neroli
Rose • Sandalwood

Sometimes I forage fennel and mugwort on my hikes, and I grow chamomile. If you can't grow your own or get them from someone you know, I recommend trying Mountain Rose Herbs (see Resources).

TO STEAM YOUR FACE:

- Thoroughly cleanse your face.
- Boil three cups of water in a pot. Remove the pot from the heat, and pour the water into a bowl.
- Add three tablespoons of a mix of herbs and flowers, and three to five drops of essential oil (if using). A little goes a long way.
- Cover and let steep for five minutes.
- Place your face over the bowl, and using a towel or cloth, create a tent to trap the steam.
- Sit for ten minutes, relaxing and visualizing beautiful images. (I like to think of being bathed in nourishing rays of light, almost as if I am under a waterfall.)
- Rinse your face with cool water.
- Follow with moisturizer or face oil.

Honoring Our Connection to the Natural World

I spent the first ten years of my life as a wilding in Iran, running through cherry groves, playing in the shadow of the Alborz Mountains, and dodging the buzz of dragonflies as I splashed in lily ponds. I felt such a bond with the natural world that simply seeing a tree cut down would leave me inconsolable for days.

Ayurveda flourished at a time when humans were more connected to the natural world around them. The rhythms of the day were more related to seasons and the cycles of human life. Modern advances have caused us to lose our essential connection with the earth, but when we make a point of seeking to regain that connection, our rhythms become more fluid and in tune with natural cycles. We can do this by spending time outdoors. If we live in a city, we can visit nearby parks and be among trees, plants,

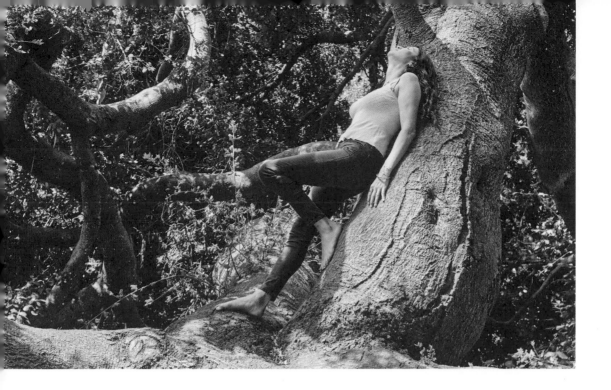

and flowers. If we live by canyons or an ocean, then we can make time each day to connect there with the source of all being. Listen to the sounds and smell the scents of nature, and honor yourself by honoring the cycles and bounty of Mother Earth.

Earthing

One way to connect with nature is simply to walk barefoot. We used to be in almost constant contact with the earth through the soles of our feet, but now we spend most of our time indoors or in shoes. Earthing is an Ayurvedic practice that many use to connect with nature. Simply going barefoot outside can help you reestablish your bond with nature. Our feet are actually portals to health, and through them, we can take in the natural minerals and enzymes of the earth. Doing so helps lower heart rate, decrease inflammation, calm the nervous system, and stimulate pressure points that can improve circulation. The Japanese even have a special term for the healing and cleansing power of nature: *shinrin-yoku*, which means "forest-bathing." Even if you can't go barefoot, taking a walk in the woods will do wonders for your whole being.

CHAPTER FOUR

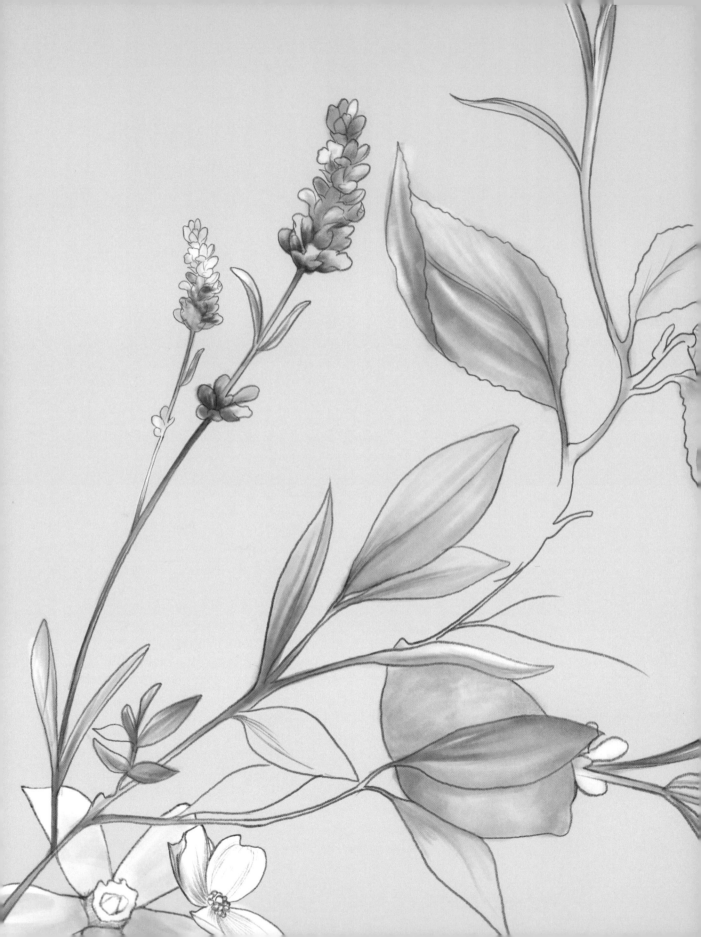

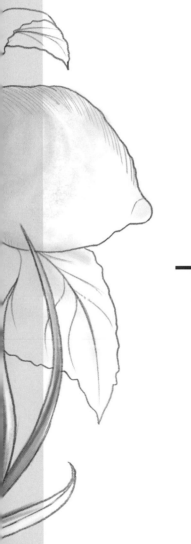

Beauty Treatments

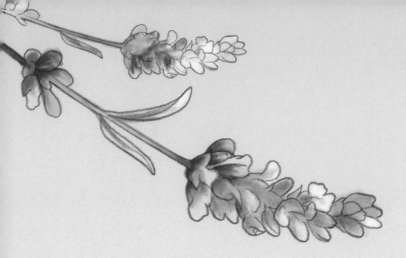

I was never one of those girls who saved up to buy the latest makeup or miracle potion. In Iran, my mother had a bottle of Chanel No. 5 and a tub of Pond's cold cream, but we were far removed from the packed aisles of a drugstore. When we moved to the United States, I brought with me an aversion to department stores and grocery stores and was drawn instead to artisans and the farmers' markets that most closely resembled the vibrant bazaars and fresh markets I'd grown up with.

Making my own products came to me quite naturally as an adult. You make your own food to be careful about what you put in your body, so why wouldn't you make your own products and treat what you put *on* your body with equal reverence and care? While conventional products may work for a short amount of time, many of them will cause harm in the long run, and I truly believe that beauty and self-care are cumulative. There is no quick fix.

Taking the time to make your own products is a way of pausing the frenetic pace of modern life. It is an act of creation that provides an experience far more personal and sensual than just unscrewing the lid of a jar. Creativity has no judgment, and it can morph into anything. You connect with the ingredients through sight, touch, smell, and taste, and as you become the alchemist of your own beauty, the flow takes over. You experiment with scents and textures, adding new elements that speak to what you need. When you are done, you hold in your hands something that will not just beautify your skin but also transform your whole being.

Now, instead of foraging flowers that grow at my feet, I am mixing sea algae from the lakes and wild rivers of Oregon, rose hips from the hills around California, and kukui nut oil from the Hawaiian tropical paradise of Kauai. Still, when I go into my studio and listen to my mantras, I am transported back to my childhood gardens, and I am in awe and filled with gratitude.

I offer you these recipes as a way to sensually indulge your skin and hair, using ingredients that you often have on hand. There is no right way to use these recipes. Doing so is a personal experience, and at the heart of these beauty rituals is allowing our intuition the space to breathe and blossom and lead us to what our bodies need.

Generally, the recipes are very safe, but use caution if you have allergies or sensitive skin. If there is anything that you think you might be allergic to or that might

cause harm, it is a good idea to test it on the inside of your arm. You can apply the oil, essential oil, or ingredient to the skin (wash it off if it is a mask component) and wait twenty-four hours to see if any irritation develops.

Make the most of this step on your wellness journey by creating some time for you; get messy and enjoy.

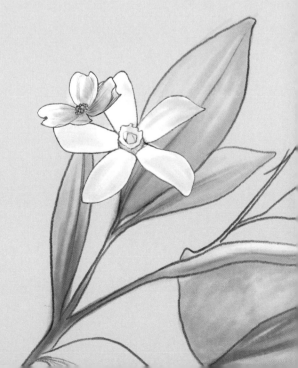

My Pantry Is My Beauty Counter

I love being able to turn to the kitchen when I need something for my skin or hair. It's inexpensive and convenient, and since the ingredients are natural and edible, they can be used without risk of damage or irritation (see page 141). I was an actress for most of my adult life, and I never thought I would do anything else—until I began making self-care products. Each one is a story, and the ingredients are the characters. The magic is in how they come together, to complement and contrast with one another. There is no right or wrong way to mix natural ingredients. You can add or subtract based on what your skin or hair needs at the moment, and to suit your preference.

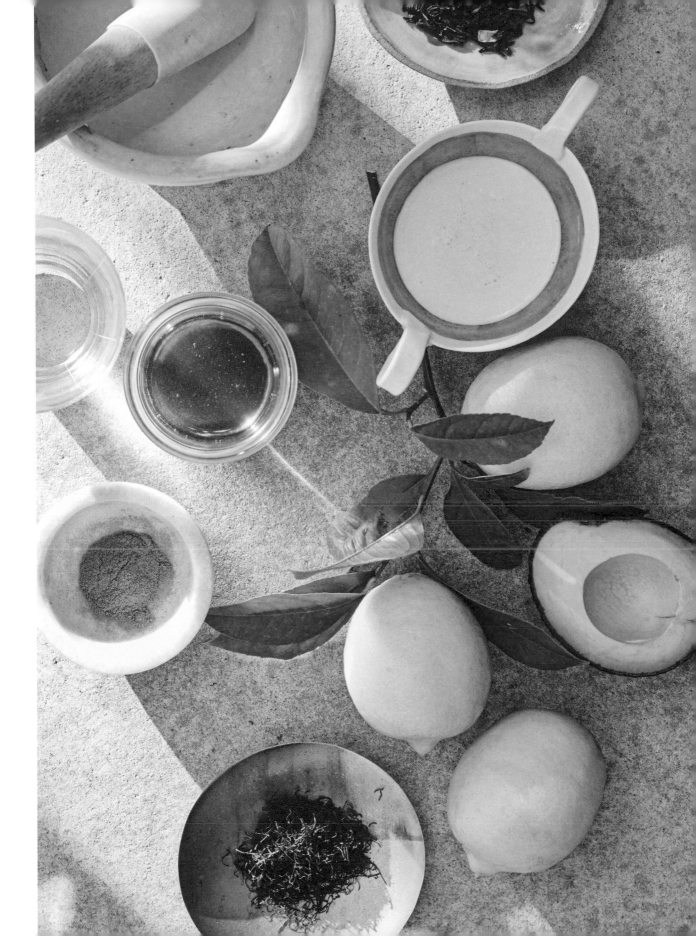

Following are the items you'll always find in my pantry.

*A note on using ingredients produced by animals:
It is always important to give gratitude—to the
industrious bees that created the honey, to the
chickens that laid the eggs. I like to pour a little of
their gift on the earth as a reminder to be grateful.*

Aloe

Most of us know aloe from using it to soothe a
sunburn, and its cooling effects come from hormones
that help heal wounds and calm inflammation. I
drink aloe juice (see page 214) from time to time
to deliver these same effects to my entire body.

Amla Fruit

This beautiful Indian fruit ripens on the tree and bursts
open in autumn. It is full of antioxidants and provides us
with so many of our nutrients. It can help skin, hair, and
hormonal balance, and it will continue to give and give.

Apple Cider Vinegar

Apple cider vinegar has been used for beauty since
ancient Roman times, and the empress of Hungary
was said to have had beautiful skin from applying
it to her face as toner. It is naturally antiseptic
and antibacterial, which makes it great for calming
acne, and it helps to balance the pH of the skin.

Avocados

Avocados are full of good fats and moisture for your
hair and skin, and your body will rejoice in soaking
them up, inside and out. The avocado is such a
dignified fruit with its beautiful emerald-green flesh
that delivers a big caress of lusciousness to your skin.

Bananas

Bananas are full of potassium, which helps to
strengthen hair, repairing damage and preventing
breakage. They are also full of powerful antioxidants
like vitamins A, C, and E and zinc, which can prevent
aging and nourish the skin.

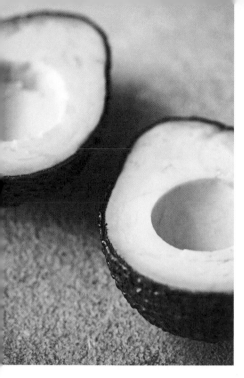

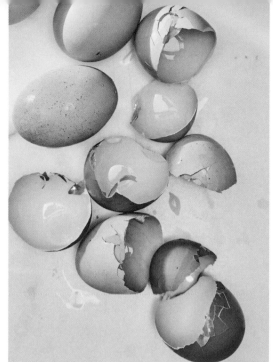

Bhringaraj

Bhringaraj symbolizes reverence for the sacred masculine. It promotes hair growth, can create lustrous hair, and also calms the nervous system.

Egg Yolks

Egg yolks are rich in sulfur content, which helps in relieving dandruff symptoms and in maintaining a healthy scalp. Eggs are a wonderful source of protein and lecithin, which aid in moisturizing and strengthening hair. Lecithin acts as a natural emulsifier, which means that it binds together the ingredients of a homemade hair mask and converts them into a homogenous mixture. I get eggs from my own chickens, Frida and Maria.

Green Tea

Green tea is rich in powerful antioxidants, and applied topically, it helps to flush toxins from the skin and reduce inflammation.

Honey

In ancient Greek myths, honey was called ambrosia, the food of the gods. The humble bees who work so

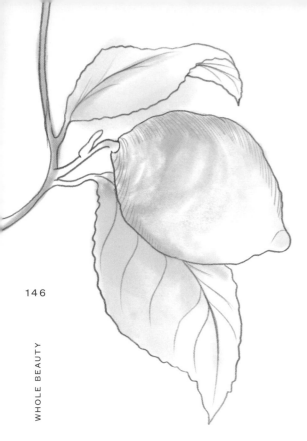

hard to create this elixir of life are always feeding us. Honey is sweet and dewy, a balm for our skin, our soul, and the planet. It's simply divine, and also antibacterial and super moisturizing, so it can help calm acne and give your skin a glow. Use raw honey, as processed honey has been stripped of its beneficial probiotics and enzymes.

Lemons

I love to drive through Ojai and smell the fresh neroli and lemon blossoms scenting the air. Bright and energetic, lemons remind me of the sun, and just a whiff of them can create that happy energy in your mind. Lemons can also serve as an excellent toner for your skin.

Nutmeg

Nutmeg is known in Ayurveda for its antiseptic and antiviral properties, which makes it great for helping to heal acne and reduce scarring.

Papaya

Called "fruit of the angels" by Christopher Columbus, papaya is full of papain enzymes, which help clear away dead cells as well as feed your skin with vitamins A, C, and E.

Pearl Powder

Pearl powder reminds me of moon dust, and yet it comes from seashells in the ocean. It feeds us with minerals that we are lacking so that we can shine like iridescent moon pearls.

Pineapple

Kauai is my land of bliss. I love to walk upon its earth and pick its exotic fruits. I especially savor the nectar of pineapple on my tongue, mashing the pulp between my fingers and feeling the juices run across my skin. Pineapple is one of many tropical fruits that are full of antioxidants and exfoliating enzymes to make you glow.

Raw Milk

Unlike pasteurized milk, raw milk still contains a lot of the good bacteria and enzymes that will feed your skin. Now more and more dairies are producing raw milk, and there are food co-ops that sell it. Finding it might take a bit of research, but it will be well worth it! If you can't find raw milk, make sure you are using organic milk that has not been treated with any hormones.

Rose

Roses are the queen of all flowers, with a higher measure of chi than any other. Mother Mary is represented by the rose, the most divine flower of all. It is wonderful for the skin, the heart, the soul, and the spirit. Rose oil, crushed rose petals, and rose hip oil are all anti-aging, moisturizing, and anti-inflammatory.

Royal Jelly

As a beekeeper, I have such a reverence for the bees. Hair can become brittle from the water and the air, and rubbing just a little bit of royal jelly—a secretion of worker bees that feeds the larvae and is full of amino acids and protein—through the strands of your hair or the roots at the scalp and allowing those precious

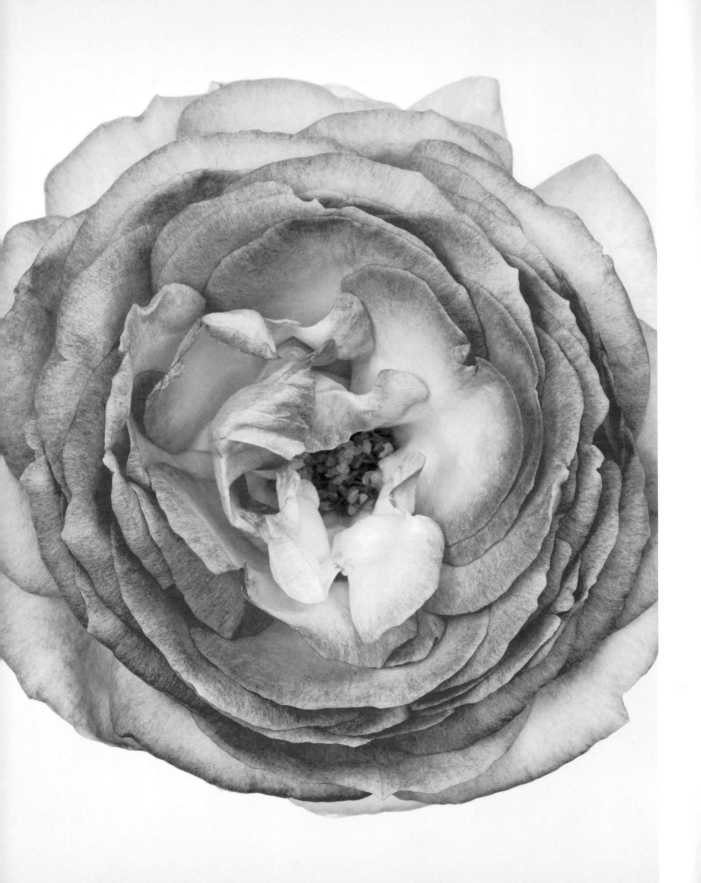

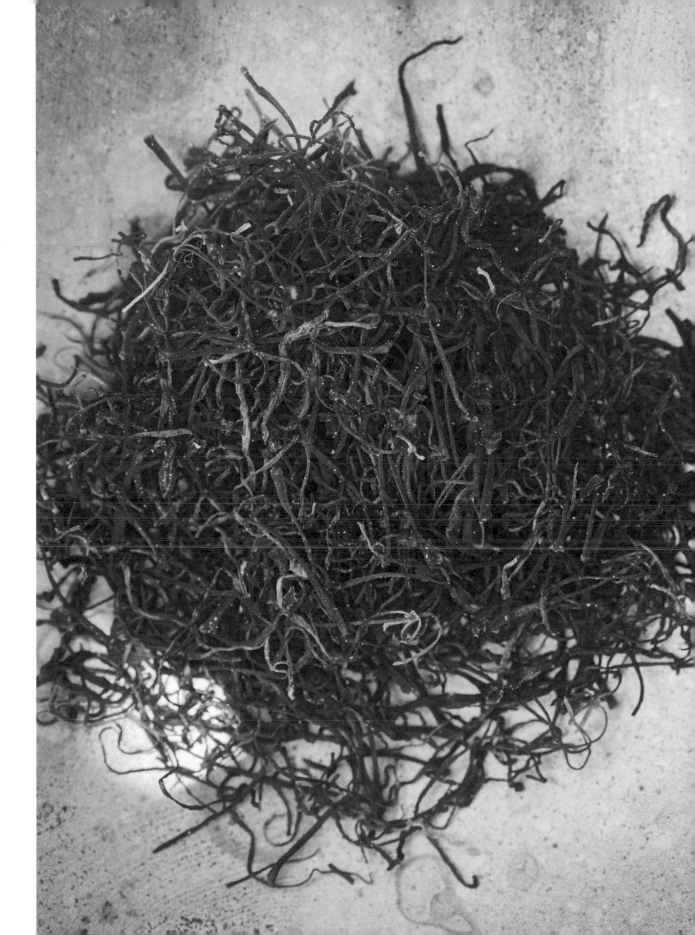

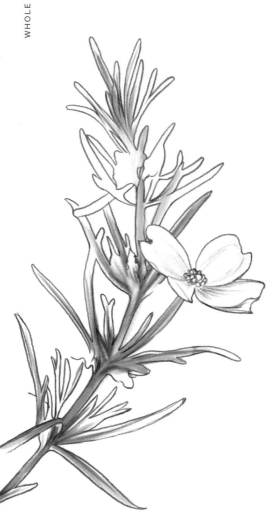

nutrients to soak in can give you luscious locks. Rich in protein; vitamins B_1, B_2, and B_6; biotin; and folic acid, royal jelly is wonderful for rejuvenating the scalp and helping to prevent prematurely gray hair.

Saffron

O saffron, you represent the nights of Persia. You smell like summer and you shine like the bright sun. Grains of white rice become a celebration when touched by your golden hue. You illuminate the face and open the heart to a feeling of endless possibility. Saffron is a magical ingredient that does wonders for clarifying the skin and evening out its tone. Just smelling a few silken red strands will awaken you to the powers of this magical ingredient.

Sandalwood Powder

Not only does sandalwood have a beautiful, uplifting scent, but it also reduces pigmentation and scarring and helps to heal blemishes.

Shatavari

Shatavari is a wonder herb from the ancient land of India that is especially good for women. It makes your hair shine and your skin glow, and it calms your hormones.

Shikakai

Shikakai is an Ayurvedic herb that is often used to cleanse the hair because of its astringent, anti-dandruff properties. It is also rich in vitamins A, C, and K, which aid in nourishing the hair.

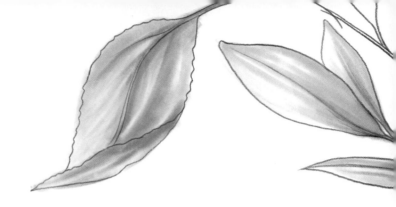

Turmeric

Turmeric is like powdered gold and sunshine. When used on the skin or taken internally, it can create optimal health and vibrancy and help heal and prevent inflammation. The wealth of the earth is given to us through turmeric.

Water

Having access to clean water should be so simple. Sadly, it is not. For those of us who are fortunate enough to live in a place where the tap water is potable, we know it is still very rarely healthy and has often been treated with chemicals such as chlorine and fluoride. When water is bottled in plastic, chemicals can leach from the packaging into the water, leading to liver and kidney stagnation and toxic buildup. It's preferable to have a water filtration system installed in your home, buy water in glass bottles, or get water directly from a spring. Mountain Valley and Castle Rock are two brands that I like, and FindASpring .com can help you locate spring water in your area.

Yogurt

Creamy yogurt is like a sweet, cooling embrace on a hot summer day. It is alive, full of beneficial enzymes and probiotics, and is a superfood for your skin. Plain yogurt contains zinc, which is anti-inflammatory and promotes cell reproduction; lactic acid, which is mildly exfoliating and great for wrinkles; calcium, which is an antioxidant and facilitates skin renewal; and B vitamins, which help keep skin glowing. You can mix yogurt with other ingredients to make a mask, or use it solo as a moisturizing treat for skin and hair.

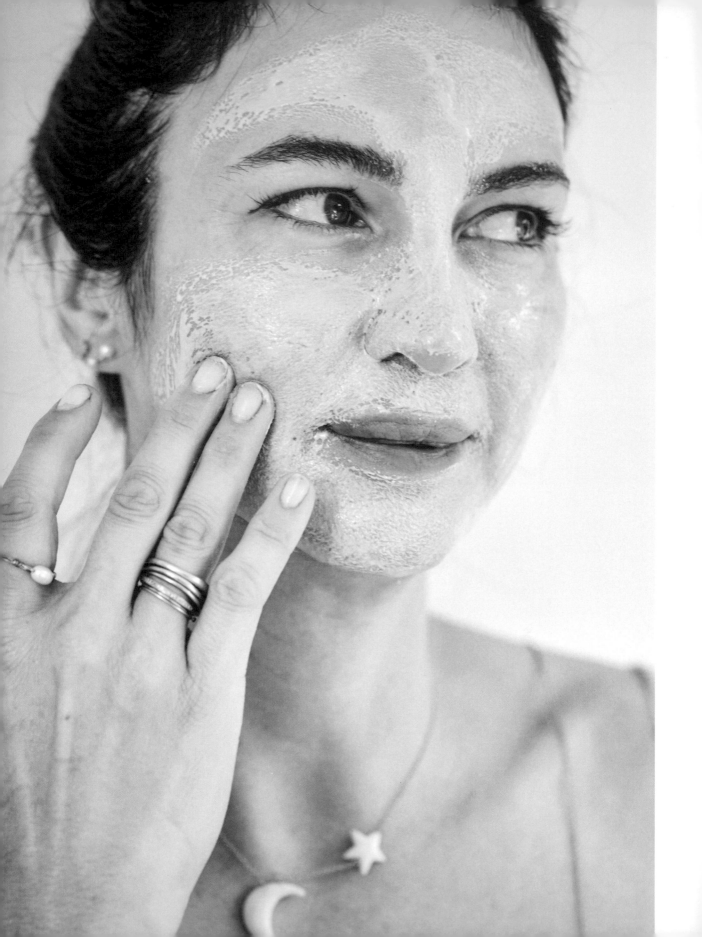

My Favorite Beauty Recipes

The beauty of the recipes in this chapter is that all you need to make them are a few kitchen items, like a blender, coffee grinder, funnel, saucepan, and whisk.

Face

We need to treat our facial skin with even more tenderness and grace than we do the skin on the rest of our body. It is even more susceptible to wrinkles and discoloration, and the skin around the eyes can be especially fragile. Because our face is what we see when we look in the mirror, and it is where we house many of our most powerful characteristics, I feel like we are honoring our entire being when we honor this one part of our body. I love getting facial treatments from professional aestheticians, but I find these do-it-yourself facial treatments to be just as healing. Feeling the ingredients mush between your fingers and smelling the spices as you stir will activate your spirit more than anything you could buy at the store. I find it wonderfully satisfying to create a sensual, beautifying experience, full of self-love, from ingredients I already have in my kitchen.

The following treatments are gentle enough that they can be used on all skin types, but each one notes which type of skin it will be most beneficial for. All of the recipes make one treatment, so feel free to double or triple them as needed to beautify with friends.

Plumping Goddess Nectar Mask

154

For
Dry and mature skin types

Recommended Use
Once a week, to feed your skin
and being

¼ cup avocado
¼ cup mashed banana
¼ cup raw honey
¼ cup plain yogurt

This mask is rich, creamy, and sensuous, full of beneficial fats that can help imbue parched skin with moisture. Caring for your skin shouldn't be a clinical process, and making this mask should be a very visceral experience. Really smoosh it around and feel it with your fingers as you're mixing it.

Using your fingers, mix the avocado, banana, honey, and yogurt in a bowl until they are well combined (the mixture should be a pale green). Wash your face and pat it dry, then slowly and lovingly apply the mixture. Leave on for 20 minutes, then rinse off with cool water.

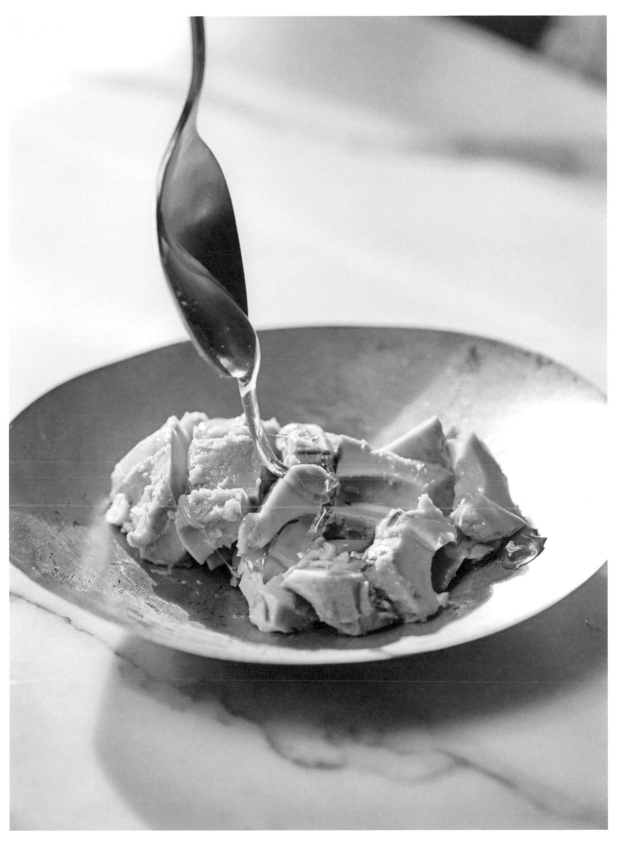

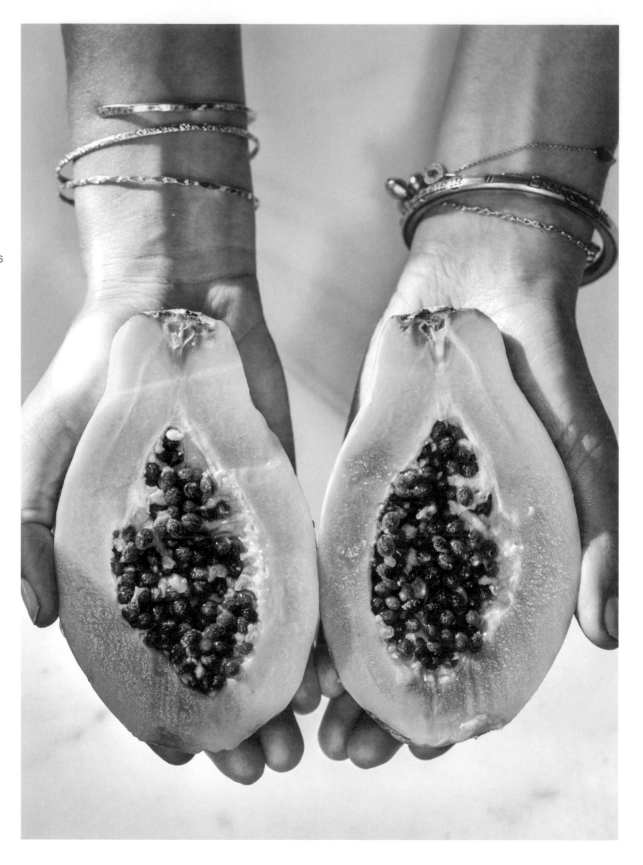

Exfoliating
Luscious Island Mask

For

All skin types, though use caution if your skin is sensitive. Natural alpha-hydroxy acids and enzymes are safer than chemicals, but they can still cause irritation.

Recommended Use

Once a month to leave your skin with a radiant glow

¼ cup papaya (see Note) or pineapple (pineapple is stronger and great to use for extra exfoliation)
¼ cup plain yogurt

I've been visiting Kauai since I was fifteen, and one of the first things I do when I land on that red, rich earth is go to the farmers' market and pick out my pineapples, papayas, mangoes, coconuts, and lychees. They don't last long in our house, but whatever we don't eat, I use to make a mask, as the acids in these tropical fruits are gentle exfoliators that help clear away dead skin. And bromelain, an enzyme that's derived from pineapples, is really good for inflammation. I love to sit with one of these masks on my face and feel my skin tingle as I bask in the feminine, Venus energy of a place ripe with beauty.

Mix the fruit and yogurt together in a bowl with a wooden spoon, using the back of the spoon to mash the fruit. It's okay if there are some chunks. Wash your face and pat it dry, then spread the mask on with your fingers. Leave on for 15 minutes, then rinse off with warm water.

Note: If you use papaya, you can also include the seeds as a potent exfoliator.

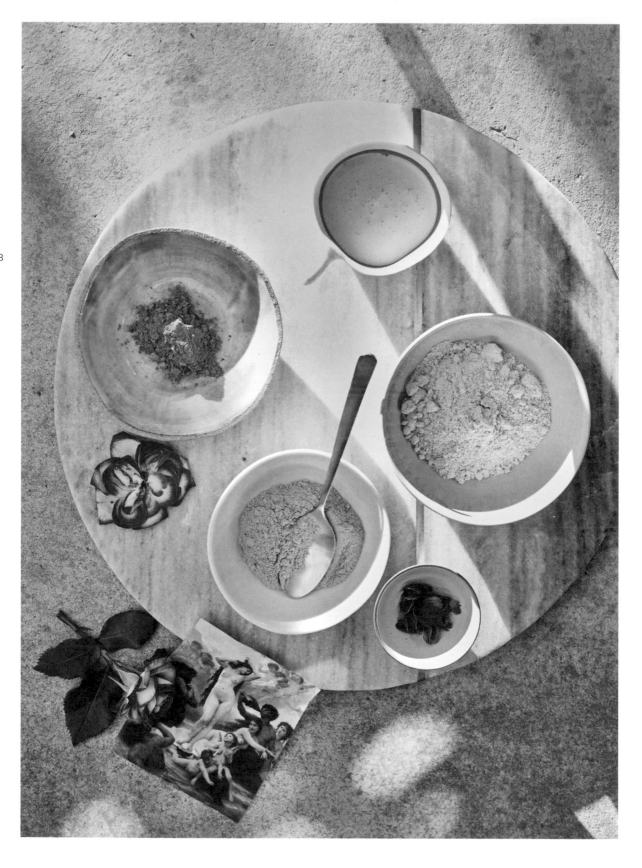

Venus
Beauty Mask

For
Normal to dry skin types

Recommended Use
Twice a month or as needed to
moisturize

5 tablespoons oat flour
3 tablespoons milk, preferably
   raw (see page 147)
1 teaspoon sandalwood powder
A small handful of crushed dried rose
   petals, plus 1 teaspoon ground

Women are ruled by Venus, who is all about
love, compassion, and prosperity. In India, she is
represented by Lakshmi. I have been honoring her
now for a few years and see signs of her popping
up in my life all the time. The scents of rose and
sandalwood instantly transport me back to the
buzzing markets in Iran. In Persian and Ayurvedic
teachings, sandalwood opens your third eye and
rose opens your heart, and this captivating fragrance
uplifts your spirits. Astringent sandalwood cools
with antibacterial properties that help prevent
acne, while rose petals deliver anti-aging moisture.
I love how beautiful and indulgent this mask feels
as it balances skin and makes it absolutely glow.

Mix the oat flour with the milk in a bowl and stir
until it forms a paste. As it does, sprinkle in the
sandalwood powder and the rose petals. Stir until you
achieve a smooth consistency. Wash your face and
pat it dry, then scoop the mask into the palm of your
hand and apply it using upward strokes. Leave on for
20 minutes, then rinse off with warm water.

Cooling Milk & Spice Mask

For
Oily and acne-prone skin types

Recommended Use
Two or three times a month, if you
have a lot of breakouts

2 or 3 whole nutmeg pods, or
    1 tablespoon ground nutmeg
1 tablespoon whole milk, preferably
    raw (see page 147), plus more
    as needed
1 teaspoon raw honey (optional;
    use only if you have exceptionally
    oily skin)

Breakouts are eruptions usually caused by too much Pitta—fire energy—in the body. We have to learn how to harness the passion and fire and put it to work for us. Otherwise, we just swallow that fire and it comes out in acne or cysts, hormonal issues. This mask treats acne by soothing and calming the skin to leave it smooth and supple. The medicinal qualities of nutmeg help to rejuvenate the skin and also treat anxiety and digestive issues in the body. Whole milk is full of nourishing fats that help moisturize, and when these two ingredients are mixed together, your skin will want to drink up the combination. (In fact, it is good enough that you *could* drink it!)

Grind the nutmeg in a coffee grinder and transfer it to a bowl. Add the milk and the honey, if using, and stir until combined to form a paste. You can add water instead of more milk to get the right consistency. Wash your face and pat it dry, then apply the mask all over or just to problem areas. You may get some tingling, but that means the mask is being activated. Leave on for 15 to 20 minutes, then rinse off with cool water.

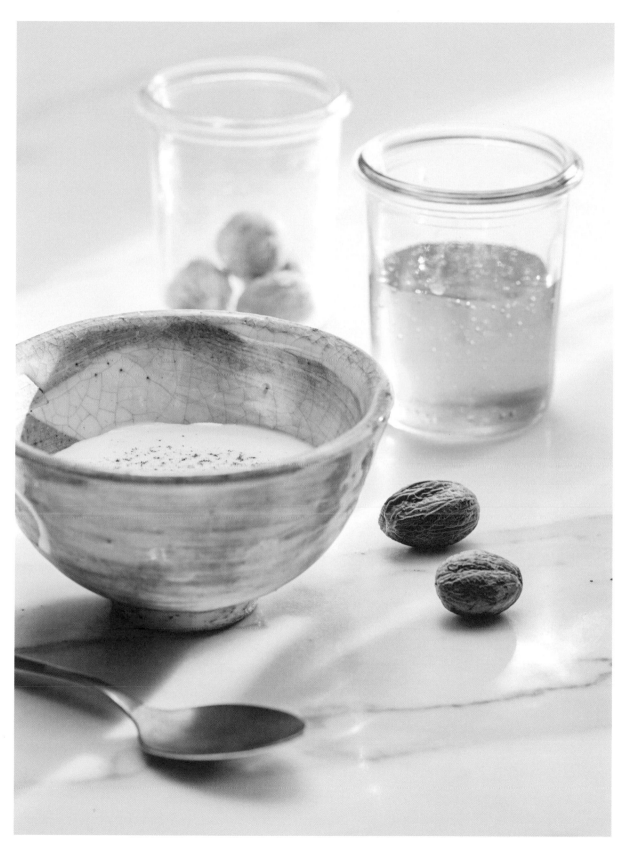

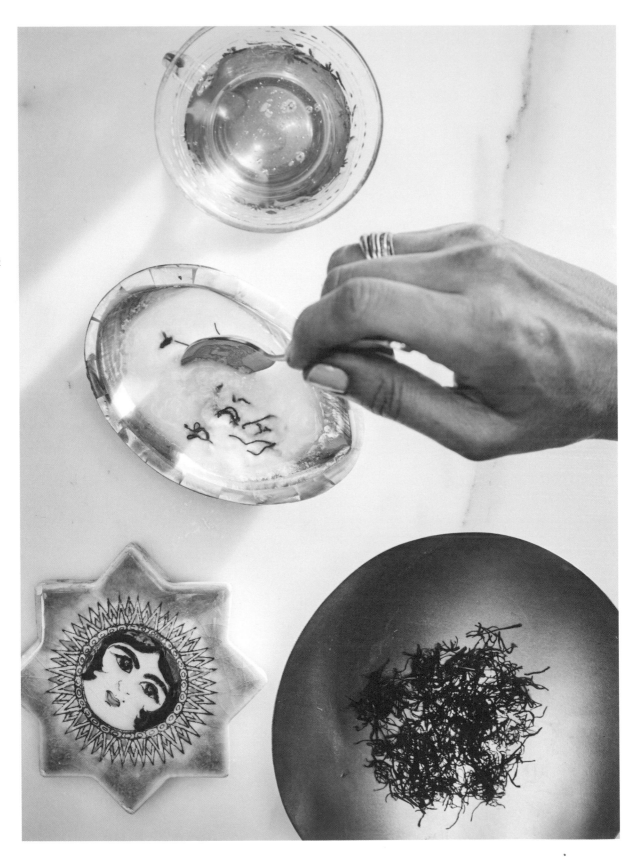

Golden
Sun Mask

For
Normal to dry skin types

Recommended Use
As needed for special occasions

½ cup plain yogurt (I prefer goat's
   or sheep's milk)
3 tablespoons raw honey
1 tablespoon saffron threads

This mask really makes you radiant, like the sun.
It combines three of my favorite ingredients—
yogurt, honey, and saffron—and it's a mix of Persian
and Ayurvedic traditions. The unusual flavor and
beautiful golden red color of saffron come from
the crocus flower, and it is said that it takes
4,500 crocus flowers to make one ounce of saffron.
Ayurvedic practices call on saffron for its incredible
healing properties in everything from reducing stress
and depression to soothing menstrual cramps and
even helping with male fertility issues. It also helps
alleviate skin discoloration, dullness, and acne. This
mask will brighten your skin for a special occasion,
birthday, holiday, or romantic date.

Combine the yogurt, honey, and saffron in a bowl and
stir until the mixture is a pale golden hue. Wash your
face and pat it dry, then brush the mask onto your
skin. Leave on for 15 to 20 minutes, then rinse off
with lukewarm water.

*Exfoliating Version: By hand, squeeze a few drops of
lemon juice into the mixture and add 1 teaspoon of
organic sugar. (I like to use coconut sugar.) Mix well
and let sit for 10 minutes before applying. Pat on,
using circular, upward motions. Leave on for 15 to
20 minutes, then rinse off with lukewarm water. Lemon
will make the mask more lightening, and sugar helps
to exfoliate.*

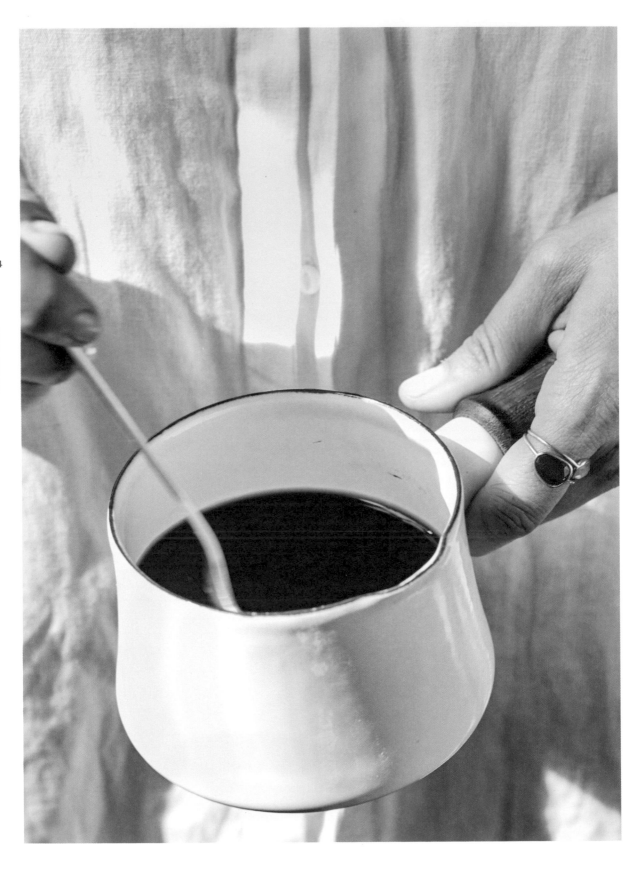

Chaga Power Mask

For
Mature or sun-damaged skin

Recommended Use
Once or twice a month

1 tablespoon chaga chunks, or
    2 tablespoons chaga powder
2 tablespoons raw honey
2 tablespoons coconut oil

The best chaga is wild-crafted in Siberia and is called "the king of medicinal mushrooms." Though it's not much to look at, chaga has more antioxidants than pomegranates and blueberries, which makes this mask like a superfood for your skin. It can help fight everything from premature aging and sun damage to broken capillaries and hyperpigmentation. You can get chaga at most health food stores, and it usually comes in raw form (chunks) or powder.

If using chaga chunks, place 1 cup water in a saucepan, drop in the chaga, and bring to a boil. Reduce the heat and let simmer for at least an hour, or until the water turns a deep reddish brown.

If using chaga powder, stir it into 1 cup boiling water, then allow to cool.

Mix the cooled chaga "tea" with the honey and coconut oil in a bowl. Wash your face and pat it dry, then apply the mask. Leave on for 15 minutes, then rinse off with lukewarm water.

Calming
Mineral Mermaid Mask

For
Oily skin

Recommended Use
Once or twice a month, or as
needed to calm breakouts

1 cup boiled green tea
   (use 2 tea bags)
1 tablespoon raw honey
1 tablespoon lemon juice
2 tablespoons agar agar

I love this mask for how smooth and hydrated it
leaves the skin. It gently exfoliates and replenishes
with much-needed minerals. Plus, it is satisfying
and fun to peel off! Agar agar is said to have been
discovered in Japan in the 1600s. It's a beautiful
binding ingredient that is derived from seaweed
and is full of iron, magnesium, copper, and calcium,
all of which make it anti-inflammatory. The honey
has the added benefit of being antibacterial.

Mix together the green tea, honey, lemon juice,
and agar agar in a saucepan and bring to a boil for
2 minutes. Remove from the heat and let sit until it
forms a thick paste. Wash your face and pat it dry,
then apply the paste and let it dry. When it has dried,
it will have a rubbery texture and you can peel it right
off. Use a washcloth and warm water to remove any
mask left on your skin.

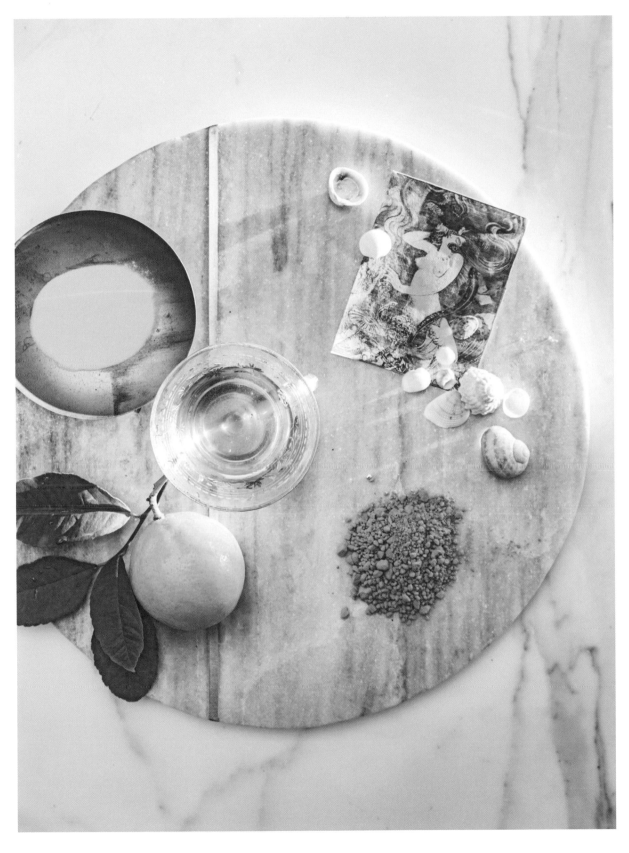

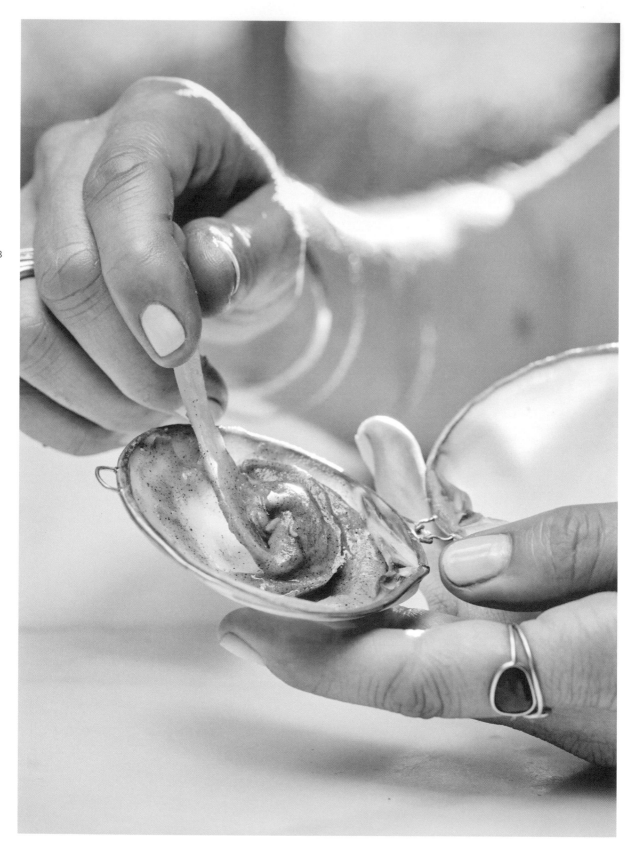

Blissful Beetroot
Lip Balm

2 tablespoons beeswax
2 tablespoons cocoa butter
2 tablespoons coconut oil
2 tablespoons beet juice or
   pureed beet

Small glass container or metal
   tin with lid

When I first began my journey into whole beauty, there were not many luxury makeup lines that were nontoxic and made with organic ingredients. Now we are incredibly lucky because that has completely changed, and there are several such makeup lines available that I love—RMS Beauty, Vapour Organic Beauty, Kosås Cosmetics, and Ilia Beauty, just to name a few (see Resources). I find this very exciting, as we can now experience vibrant and rich colors without sacrificing our health. However, when you have glowing, dewy skin, you do not need much makeup—just a reddish-pink lip tint and a light coat of mascara will do.

In a small saucepan, melt the beeswax, cocoa butter, and coconut oil over low heat until liquefied. Remove from the heat and whisk in the beet juice or puree. Put the mixture in a blender and blend on high for 30 seconds to emulsify. Transfer the mixture to the container and refrigerate until solid. The lip balm can be kept at room temperature away from direct heat or sunlight for 3 to 4 months or stored in the refrigerator for up to a year.

Tip: This lip balm will melt easily, so be careful about leaving it in your purse on a hot summer day.

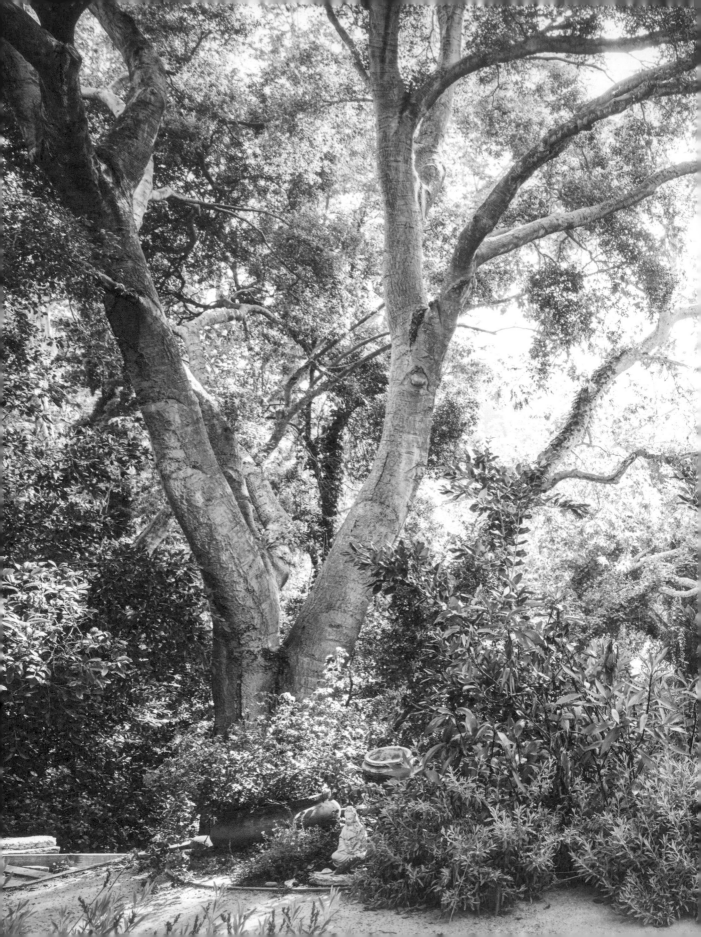

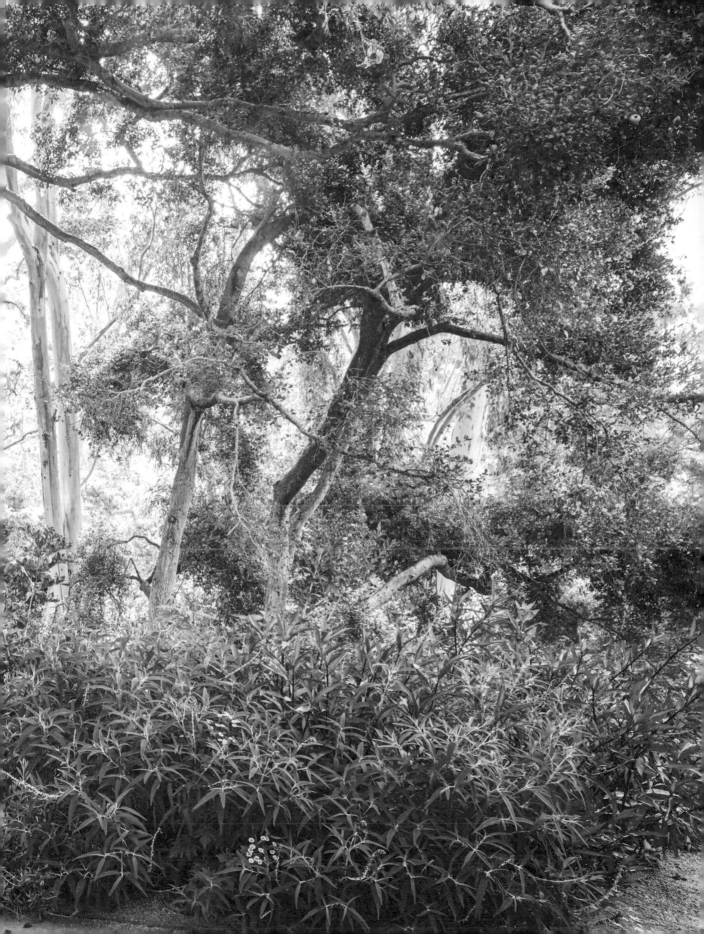

Hair

There is a story that always comes to mind when I think about hair. Legend has it that during the Vietnam War, the CIA recruited Native Americans because they were known for their remarkable ability to track animals in even the densest vegetation.

However, once the trackers got to Vietnam, they weren't able to do their work at all. They had lost all of their ability. Why? Because the government had forced them to cut their hair, and with their hair went their power.

I do believe that our hair is connected to our intuition. Our hair is both our antennae and our tail, and a strong communicator. From the Kundalini perspective, the hair is a vibrant source of creative life force that helps to funnel powerful sun energy into the frontal lobes of the brain. Your hair's health, much like your skin's, can alert you to changes in your overall health—specifically hormonal imbalances, thyroid issues, and toxicity buildup—before symptoms are manifested elsewhere in your body.

From goddesses to queens, women have always used their hair to express themselves and their intentions. Whether it's Jean Seberg's pixie cut, Goddess Lalita's thick, dark locks scented with champaca flowers, or Cleopatra's blunt-cut bangs, hair is a source of feminine power, and keeping yours healthy and lustrous will also help your aura shine. Use these treatments to deep-condition your hair before shampooing and conditioning as you normally do.

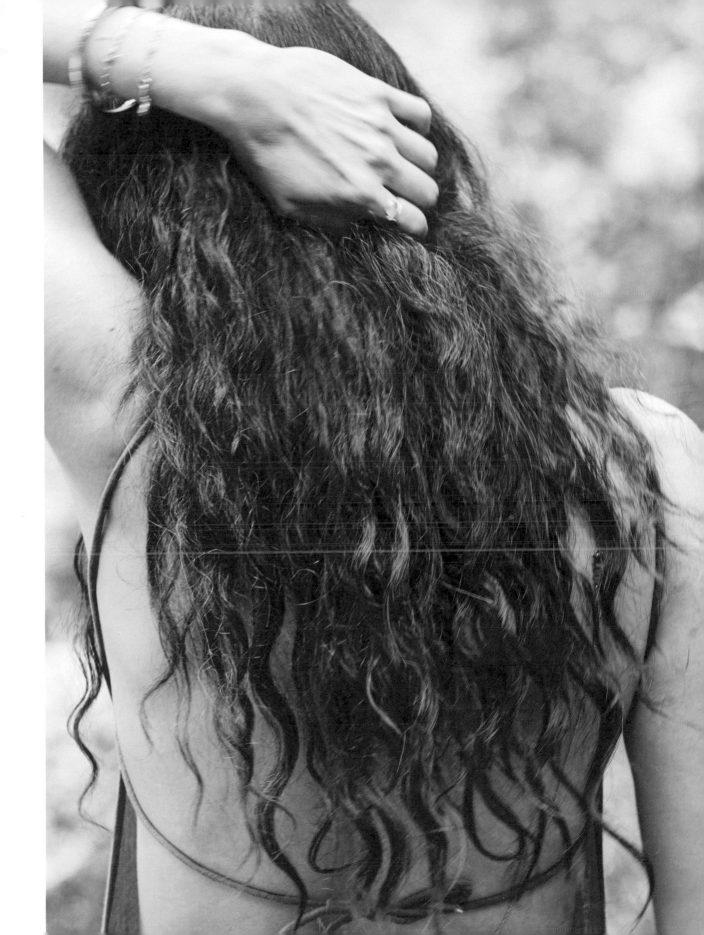

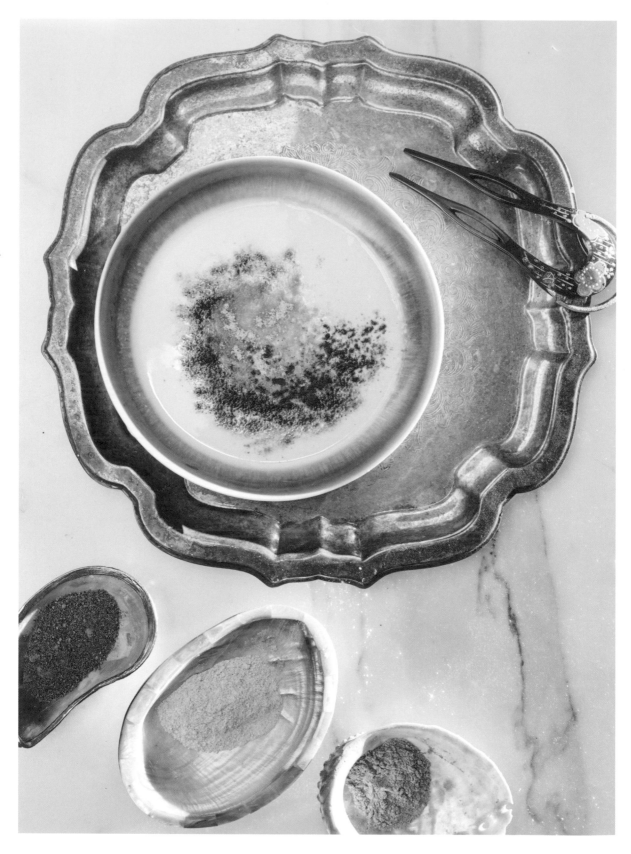

Lustrous Lakshmi Mask

For
All hair types

Recommended Use
Once a month

1 tablespoon fenugreek powder
1 tablespoon shikakai powder
2 tablespoons amla fruit powder
2 tablespoons plain yogurt

Named for the Hindu goddess of fortune and prosperity, this mask adds some love to your locks as it conditions, stops dandruff, and makes your hair grow longer, stronger, and faster. It's a tridosha mask. Fenugreek seeds are an Indian spice known for their sweet smell and helpfulness in treating hair loss and baldness. Shikakai powder comes from a common Asian shrub and is high in antioxidants like vitamins A, C, and K. It helps to balance the pH of the hair and make it shiny. Amla fruit has three times more vitamin C than an orange. It nourishes hair from the scalp to the ends. If you are having trouble finding these herbs in your area, you can order them from Banyan Botanicals or Dual Spices (see Resources).

Soak the powders in water (5 or 6 tablespoons should be enough, but add as much as you need to thoroughly wet the powders into a pastelike consistency) in a bowl for a few hours. Stir in the yogurt and let sit for an hour. Apply to your hair and scalp. Leave on for an hour, then lightly shampoo.

Apple Cider Vinegar Rinse

For

All hair types

Recommended Use

Once a month, as a nice reset for the hair

1 tablespoon apple cider vinegar (I love Bragg and Fire Cider)

8 ounces water

A few drops of an essential oil, such as rosemary or lavender, to stimulate the scalp and help mask the pungent scent of the vinegar

Glass jar, cup, or spray bottle

You'll be amazed at how soft and shiny your hair can be when you rinse it with apple cider vinegar, which acts as a detoxifier. The acidity of apple cider vinegar helps to balance the pH of your hair, and it also strips off the residue left by traditional hair products, leaving the hair unbelievably silky. It has zero harmful chemicals and a price tag far lower than anything you could buy at a salon.

Combine the vinegar, water, and essential oil in the jar, cup, or spray bottle and stir or shake to mix well. Pour over or spray through clean, wet hair. Leave it on for 1 to 2 minutes, then really rinse it out. If you like, apply a traditional conditioner on your ends afterward.

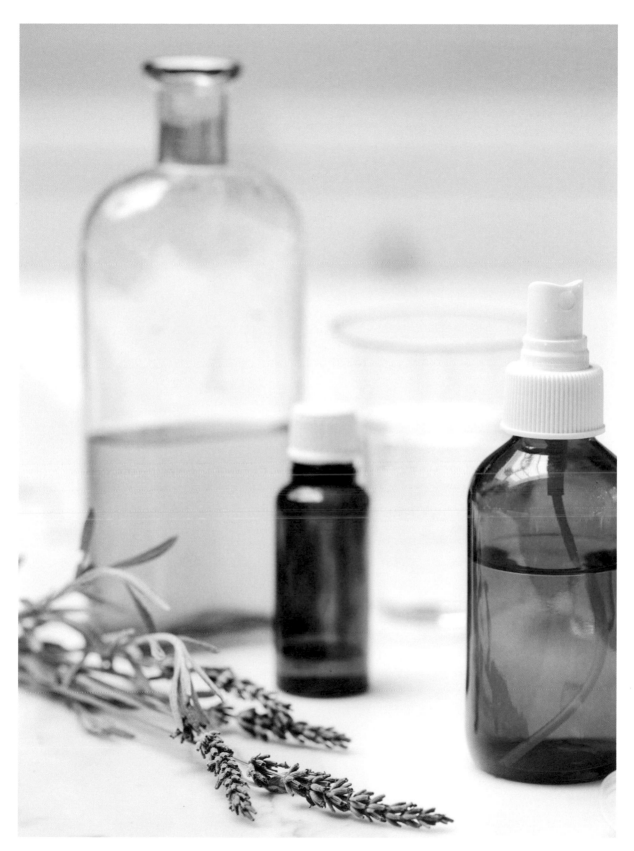

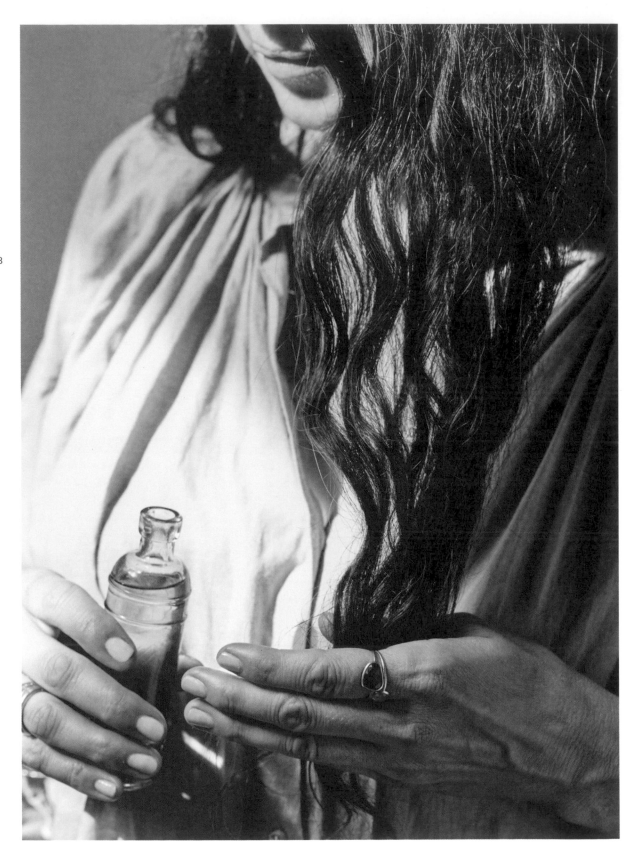

Powerful
Locks Mask

For
Those with thinning hair

Recommended Use
Once or twice a month

2 to 3 teaspoons bhringaraj oil
2 to 3 ounces coconut or almond
  oil (depending on the length of
  your hair)

As they age, many women experience a decrease in thyroid production. This affects the level of testosterone their bodies produce, which can in turn affect hair growth and thickness. This mask helps to stimulate hair growth and can also give your mane a boost if you have hair loss after pregnancy. In Ayurveda, bhringaraj, one of the main ingredients in this recipe, is known as the "king of hair" for how well it promotes hair growth, reduces balding, and stops premature graying.

In a bowl, mix the bhringaraj oil and coconut or almond oil with enough warm water to form a thick paste. Cover the scalp with the paste, then massage the oil through the hair, from the scalp down to the ends. Leave on for 20 minutes, then lightly shampoo.

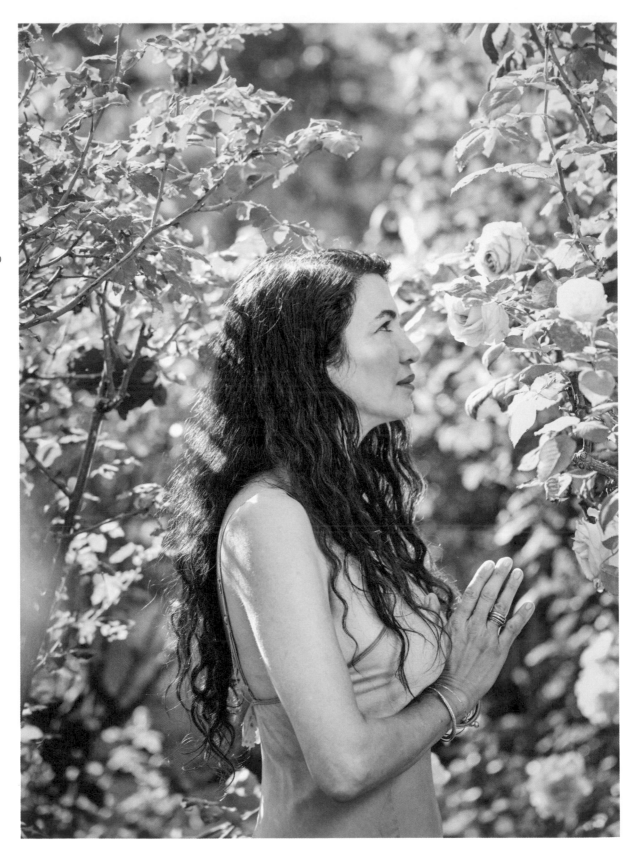

Silky Tresses Mask

For

Dry, dull, or damaged hair. Also great to use if you regularly straighten or blow-dry your hair.

Recommended Use

Once a month

1 banana
1 egg yolk
2 tablespoons raw honey
1 tablespoon olive oil (optional; use only if you have dry hair)

Egg yolks are rich in fat and protein. They moisturize, fight frizz, and leave hair gleaming. You can put egg yolk directly on your hair for a quick shine boost, or make this simple mask with enzyme-rich honey to also help thicken your hair and leave it gorgeous and bouncy. I love to imagine the golden rich yolk of the egg penetrating and seeping into my being as a healing golden serum.

Puree the banana in a blender (or give it a good mash with your hands), then transfer to a bowl. Fold in the egg yolk, honey, and olive oil (if using). Apply to the hair, starting at the scalp and working down to the ends. Leave on for 20 minutes, then wash out with your favorite shampoo. You may follow with conditioner if you like.

Simple Shampoo

For
All hair types

Recommended Use
As often as you typically shampoo

¼ cup coconut milk
¼ cup liquid castile soap
  (I like Dr. Bronner's)
20 drops of rosemary or
  peppermint essential oil
½ teaspoon olive or almond oil

Glass jar with stopper

Most traditional shampoos foam up because they are full of sulfates, which can irritate your skin (as you well know if you've ever gotten shampoo in your eyes!) and strip your hair of much-needed moisture. This nontoxic shampoo is easy to make. Store it in a glass jar and it will last for a couple of months. You'll also find that the healthier your hair becomes, the less often you'll need to shampoo.

Combine the coconut milk, soap, essential oil, and olive oil in the glass jar. Shake well before each use, and shampoo as you normally would.

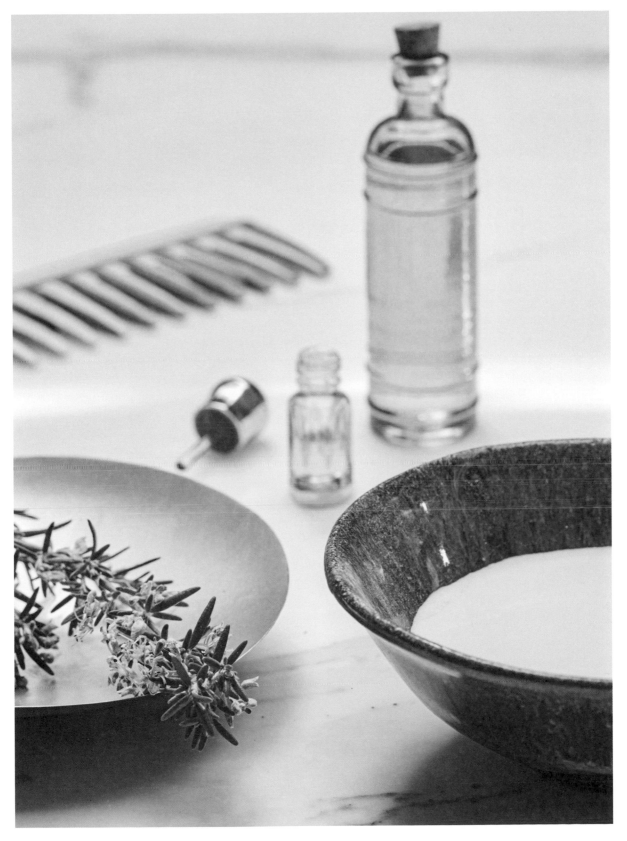

Gracious &
Divine Moisture Mask

For
Dry to normal hair

Recommended Use
Once a month

½ avocado
3 tablespoons olive oil
½ cup plain yogurt

Olive trees are some of my favorite trees, because they're so ancient and possess a beautiful simplicity; they look equally at home in the hills of Tuscany or the backyards of California. Just as the earth dries out, we as women can also—stress and depleted diets leaving us brittle. When faced with stressful situations, we crack and break instead of bending with flexibility. This mask helps to replenish us with much-needed moisture so that we can be like the olive branch—supple, abundant, and a messenger of peace. Olive oil is high in fat and oleic acid, which is wonderful for your skin as well as your hair, helping to nourish the strands from the inside out.

In a bowl, mash the avocado, then mix in the olive oil and yogurt, stirring until smooth and creamy. Apply to the hair, starting at the scalp and working down to the ends. Leave on for 20 minutes, then lightly shampoo.

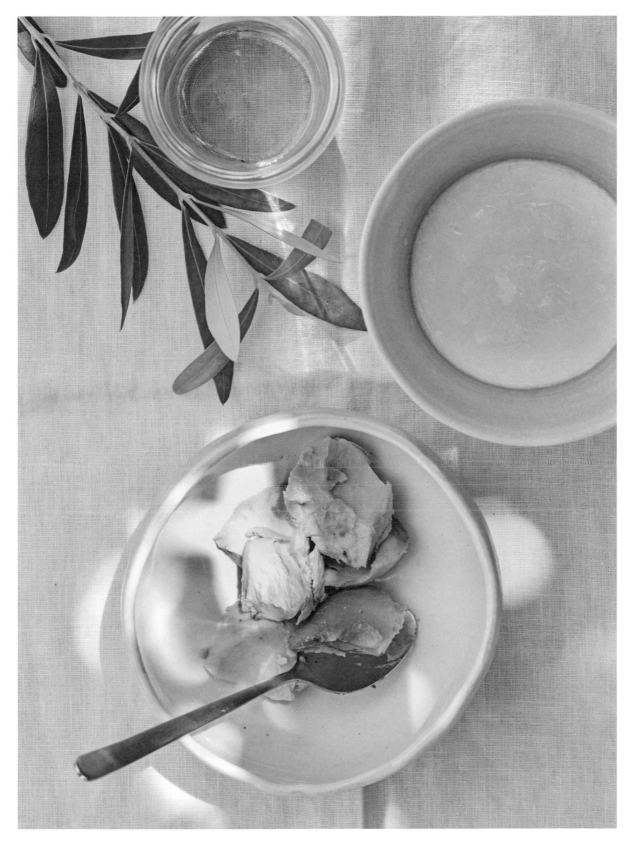

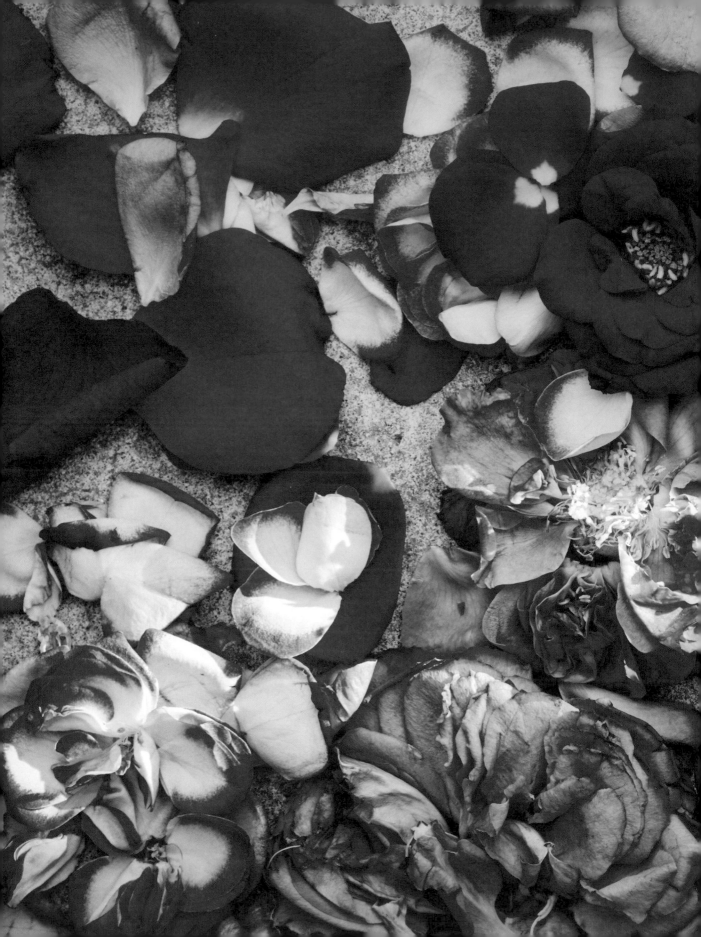

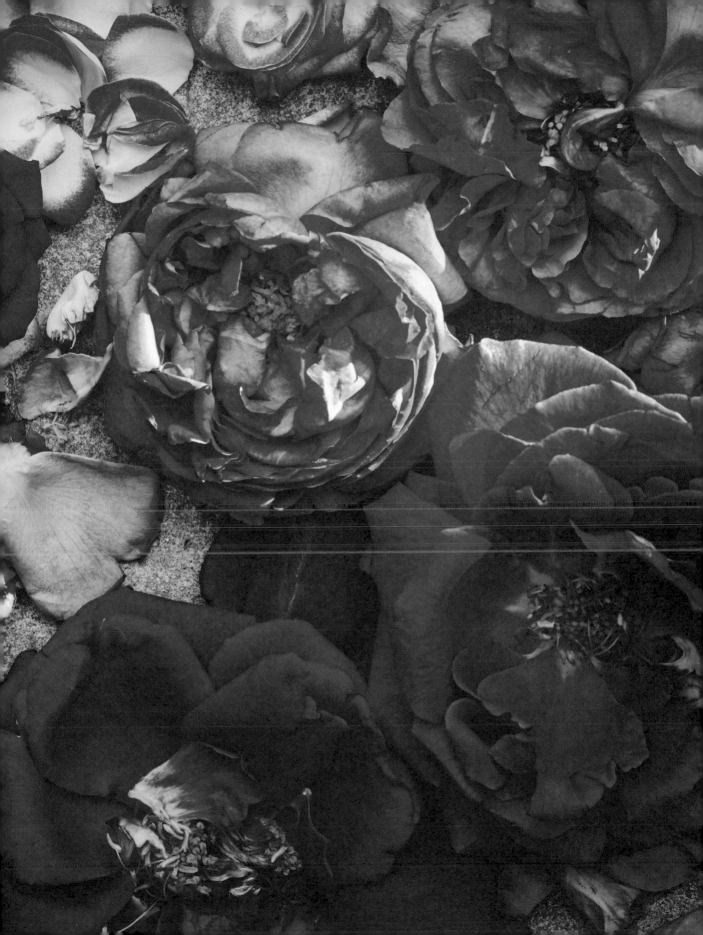

Face & Body Exfoliants

I first created my Sea Siren Scrub when camping with several women on Washington State's Orcas Island, a mystical place that inspired in me a gratitude for nature and all the wonderful women in my life. I mixed a scrub with coconut oil, shea butter, lemongrass, and a little bit of sugar, and we all spread it on our bodies and went into a sauna that had been built in the woods. I felt that we were connecting to the magical animals that give the island its name. We created a ritual around the moment, imagining ourselves as mermaids in tune with the whales. Whenever I use a scrub, I like to imagine that I am releasing what I don't need, taking off a layer of old living so that I can open myself up to letting in more sunshine and new light.

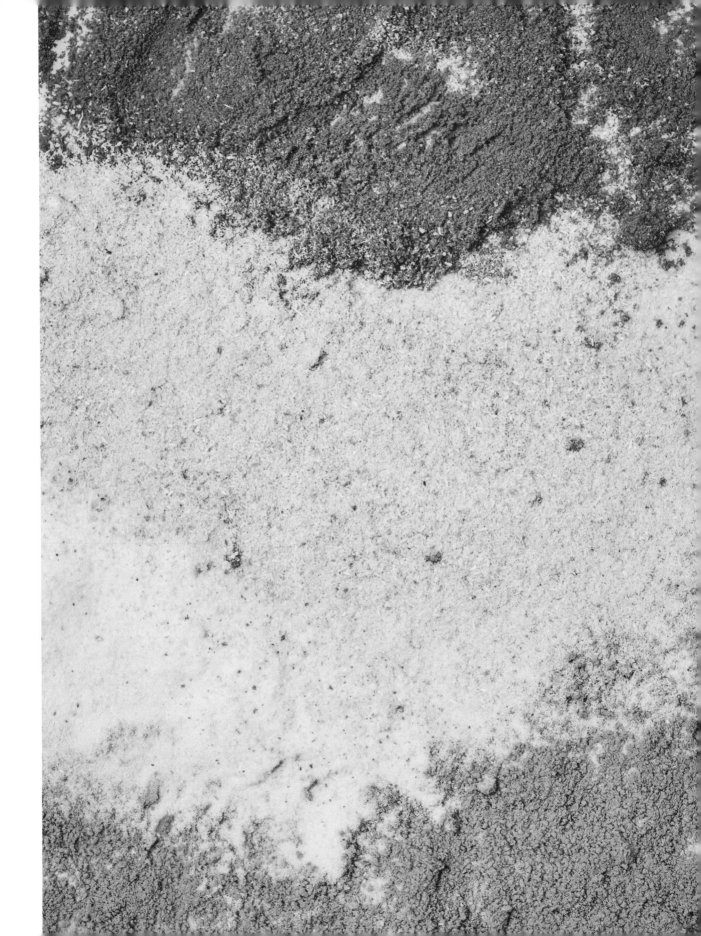

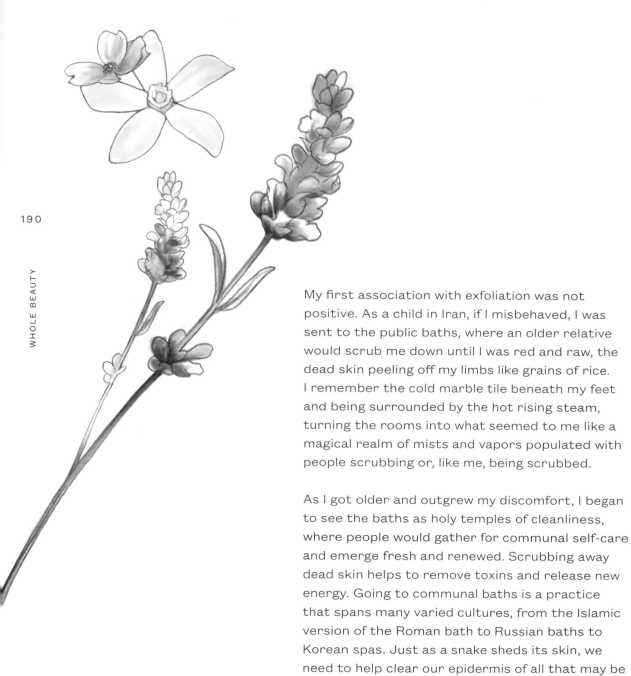

My first association with exfoliation was not positive. As a child in Iran, if I misbehaved, I was sent to the public baths, where an older relative would scrub me down until I was red and raw, the dead skin peeling off my limbs like grains of rice. I remember the cold marble tile beneath my feet and being surrounded by the hot rising steam, turning the rooms into what seemed to me like a magical realm of mists and vapors populated with people scrubbing or, like me, being scrubbed.

As I got older and outgrew my discomfort, I began to see the baths as holy temples of cleanliness, where people would gather for communal self-care and emerge fresh and renewed. Scrubbing away dead skin helps to remove toxins and release new energy. Going to communal baths is a practice that spans many varied cultures, from the Islamic version of the Roman bath to Russian baths to Korean spas. Just as a snake sheds its skin, we need to help clear our epidermis of all that may be clogging it so that it can breathe and feel alive.

In Iran, women used a *kiseh*, which is a loofah-like cloth, with *sefidab* ("white water"), a hardened chunk of minerals mixed with sheep fat, to keep their skin soft and glowing. Those can be hard to find in many parts of the world, but variations on Ayurvedic cleansing

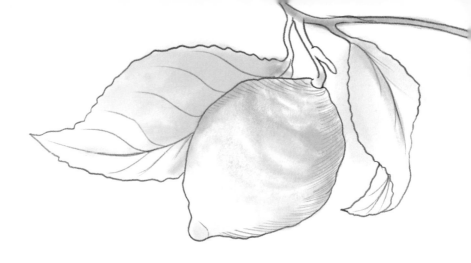

powders, called *ubtans*, are easy to make at home and provide the same benefits. Many store-bought exfoliants contain plastic microbeads, which do not decompose and remain in our rivers and oceans after they are washed down the drain. Chances are you already have many ingredients in your kitchen that can be used as natural exfoliants that won't harm your skin or the environment, such as those listed below.

Brown Rice
Brown rice is full of antioxidants, and it becomes a gentle exfoliant when you grind it uncooked in a coffee grinder until it has the consistency of rough flour.

Cane Sugar
Sugar has smaller granules than salt, which means it is gentler on your skin than a salt scrub, and it is a natural source of glycolic acid, which helps remove dead skin cells.

Chickpea Flour
Chickpea flour absorbs extra oil, and is used in Ayurveda to lighten sun damage and even skin tone.

Oat Flour
Oats have been used for centuries to calm skin irritations, and oat flour is an extremely gentle exfoliant for sensitive skin.

Blushing Bride Chickpea Face Mask

For
Normal to oily skin

Recommended Use
Once a week

5 tablespoons chickpea flour
1 tablespoon plain yogurt
¼ teaspoon turmeric
½ teaspoon sandalwood powder

Chickpea flour is wonderful in a mask, because it brightens, exfoliates, and draws out impurities from the skin. In India, brides use a chickpea mask as part of their wedding preparation ritual because it makes the skin look so young and healthy. You can buy chickpea flour at a health food store, or make your own by grinding dried chickpeas in a coffee grinder until you get a fine, fairly uniform consistency. In this mask, the turmeric has melatonin-inhibiting enzymes that help lighten scars and discoloration. Using this mask is a great way to pamper yourself before special occasions.

In a bowl, mix the chickpea flour with enough water to form a paste. Then add the yogurt, turmeric, and sandalwood powder. Wet your face and apply the mask in a circular motion. Leave on for 15 minutes, then wash off with warm water.

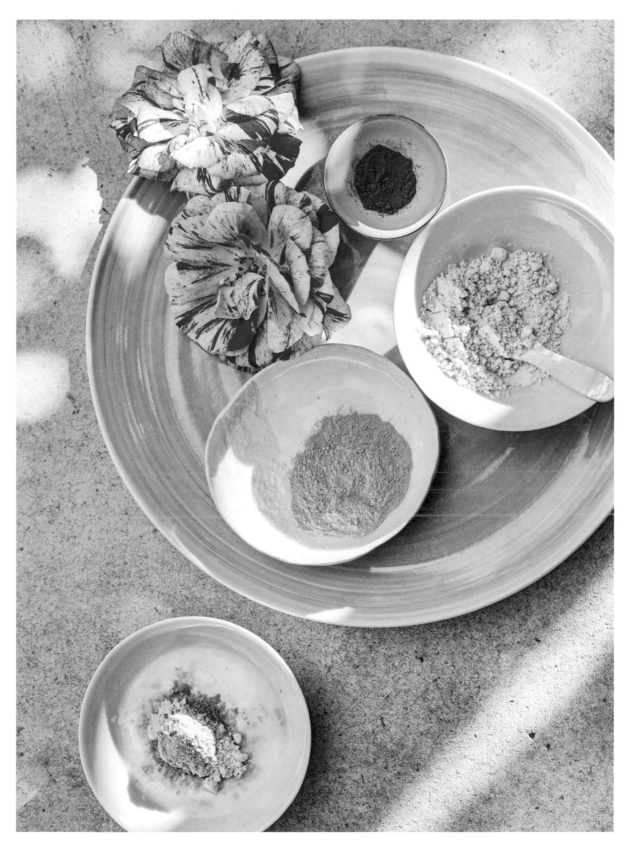

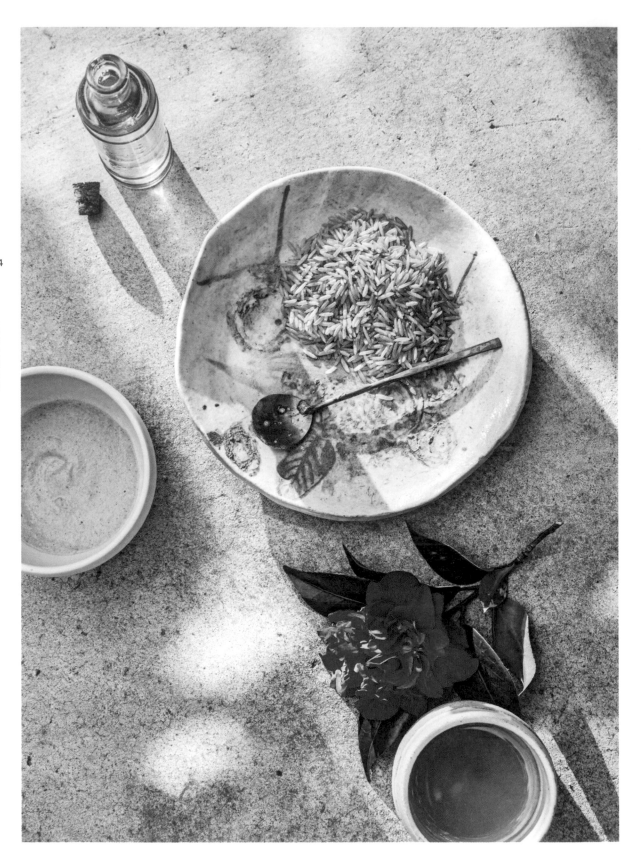

Heavenly Light
Face Scrub

For
Normal to dry skin

Recommended Use
Once a month, or whenever you feel
your skin needs exfoliation

2 tablespoons uncooked brown rice
Contents of 1 tea bag of green tea
1 tablespoon sesame seed oil

Sesame seeds are used often in Ayurvedic recipes
for their high mineral content and conditioning
aspects. Here, zinc-rich sesame oil is combined
with brown rice to slough off dead skin cells; green
tea provides a dose of anti-aging antioxidants.
Use this scrub to remove the blockage of dull cells
and reveal fresh new ones so that your skin casts a
beautiful glow.

Grind the rice and tea to a fine powder in a coffee
grinder and transfer to a bowl. Stir in the sesame
oil. Wet your face and apply the scrub in a circular
motion. Leave on for 20 minutes, then wash off with
warm water.

Revitalizing
Body Scrub

For
All skin types

Recommended Use
Once a week, or as needed

1 cup organic cane sugar
¼ cup coconut oil
¼ cup sunflower or almond oil
A few drops of vanilla essential oil
Modifications to your liking
   (optional, at right)

Mason jar with lid

I like to think of this as a "Choose Your Own Adventure" treatment. The sugar and oil base makes a wonderful scrub on its own, but you can also modify it with additional ingredients to really target your skin type or just to make it more playful and delicious. Keeping a batch ready to go in a mason jar can add a little extra splendor to your shower on even the busiest days.

Combine the cane sugar, coconut oil, sunflower oil, essential oil, and your choice of modifications, if using, in the lidded mason jar and shake well to mix. Wet your skin and apply the scrub starting at the feet, always working upward and inward toward the heart. Concentrate on rough spots like knees and elbows. Rinse well, but to preserve the moisturizing properties, do not wash off with soap.

Modifications
- For a tropical scrub, add ½ papaya, pureed
- To target dry, midwinter skin (and make your bathroom smell like the holidays), add 1 cup coffee grounds and 1 teaspoon cinnamon
- For extra brightening, add the juice of 1 lemon and 2 tablespoons raw honey
- To nourish sensitive skin, add 1 cup uncooked oatmeal and 2 tablespoons raw honey
- To target feet and elbows, add the zest and juice of 1 lemon
- For extra moisturizing, add a mashed banana

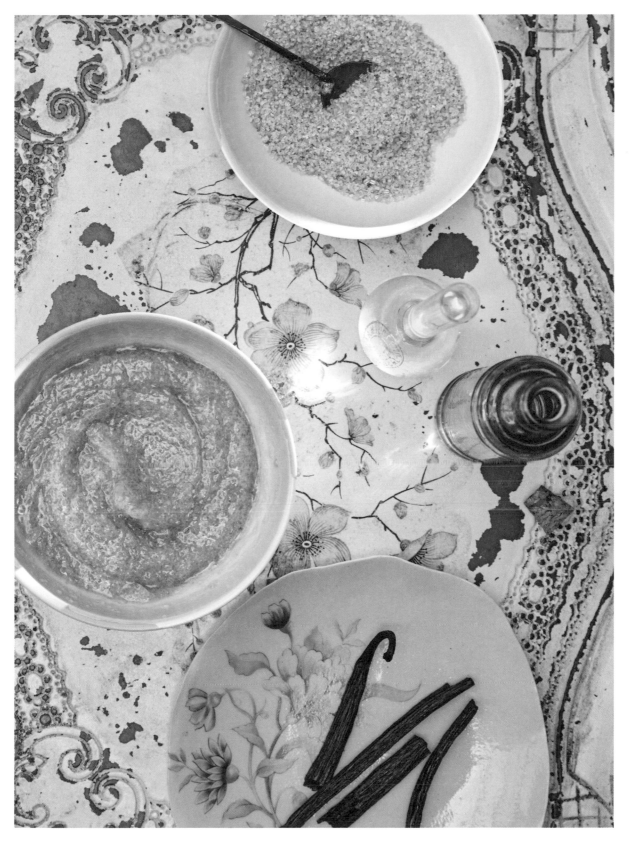

Oils for Hair, Face & Body

It might seem counterintuitive to put oil on your skin, but it's actually something your skin really needs. Just like shampoo strips the hair, most conventional cleansers strip the skin of its essential moisture. This affects the pH and microbiome of your skin, leaving it vulnerable to irritation and breakouts and speeding up the aging process. Because they are lipophilic—or fat loving—oils pass through the lipid layer of the skin faster than water-based moisturizers. The right oils will wake up your skin, soothe it, and help it glow.

Oil has devotional properties and has been used for centuries to anoint royalty. To use oils is to connect with the divine. Take a moment to savor the act of putting drops of it into your bath, the feeling of it being absorbed into your skin, of it being taken in through your hair and hands.

When using any oil, remember to take the time and intention to anoint yourself rather than just slather it on, so that you fully experience how luxurious oils can be. As with anything you are using on your skin or scalp for the first time, you may want to test for sensitivity by applying it to a small area of your inner arm, then waiting twenty-four hours to see if an irritation develops.

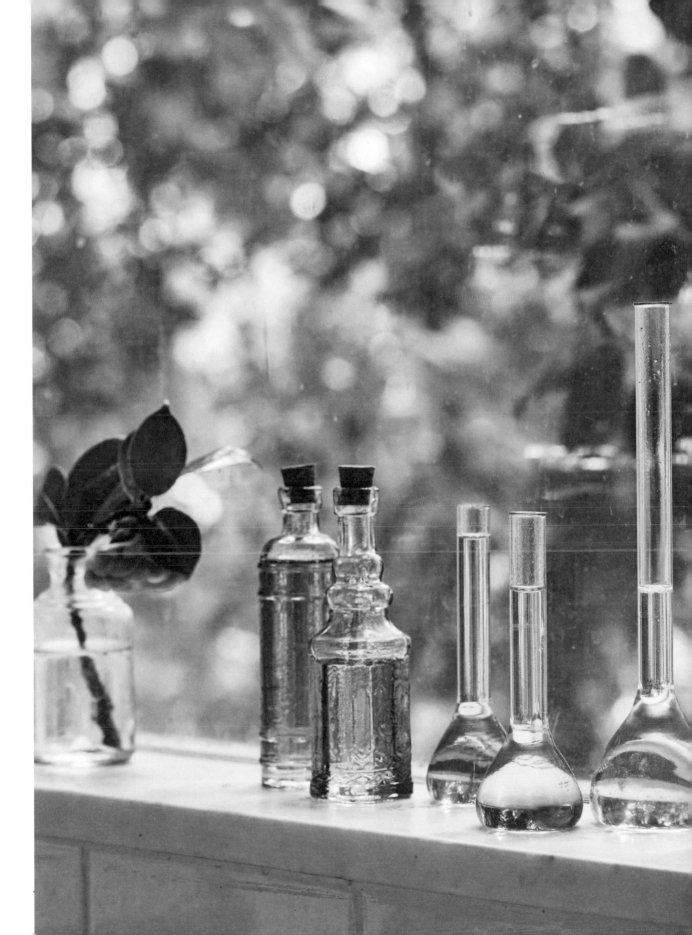

I like to have a variety of oils on hand to meet different skin and hair needs. All of these can be used alone or blended.

Almond Oil

Almond oil has been used by Ayurvedic practitioners for centuries. It is brimming with vitamin E, and massaging it on the skin below the eyes will help reduce dark circles.

Argan Oil

Argan oil is loaded with omega-6 fatty acids, linoleic acid, and vitamins A and E. It helps boost cell production and is anti-inflammatory, which is why it was historically used to treat bug bites and skin irritation.

Camellia Oil

Camellia oil is sometimes known as tea seed oil, because it comes from *Camellia sinensis*, the tea plant. It is mildly astringent, anti-inflammatory, and high in antioxidants, just like green tea.

Castor Oil

I use castor oil on my eyebrows and eyelashes, as it stimulates hair to grow back thicker and fuller. Using a clean mascara wand, I brush some on every night before bed. You can add it to your conditioner to help promote thicker hair.

Coconut Oil

Not only is coconut oil delicious, but it is also a rich, wonderful moisturizer for skin and hair, and it can be used to remove makeup. Coconut oil is rich in fatty acids and lauric acid, which is antifungal and antibacterial. It solidifies at room temperature, so when using coconut oil for masks, I usually recommend melting it in a small bowl set in warm water.

Jojoba Oil

I love to use jojoba oil as a base for face moisturizers. Native Americans use it to treat bruises and sores, and it is rich in iodine, which makes it antibacterial.

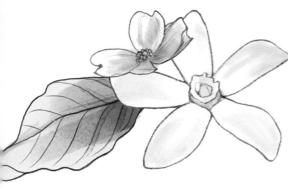

Kukui Nut Oil

A natural moisturizer that Hawaiian mermaids have been using for centuries, kukui nut oil is a sun worshipper's dream. It helps reduce sun damage and also lightens stretch marks and treats scars.

Rose Hip Oil

Rose hip oil comes from wildflowers in the Himalayas and is high in vitamins A and C. It is a powerful anti-aging oil that was used by Greek goddesses as part of their daily skin-care regimen.

Sea Buckthorn Oil

Sea buckthorn is a shrub that grows in Europe and Asia and has long been used in Russia to help protect skin against frigid winters. It heals wounds, reduces inflammation, and helps build proteins in the skin.

Sesame Oil

Sesame oil has been used for thousands of years, is mentioned in the Vedas, and is known as the "queen of the oils." Sesame seeds are rich in zinc, which is a potent antioxidant necessary for producing collagen and retaining skin elasticity.

Shea Butter

A hydrating, rich, nourishing and grounding, skin-regenerating, tridosha moisturizer that helps to stimulate collagen production, shea butter will melt into an oil with the heat from your hands.

Sunflower Oil

Sunflower oil is a great base for body oils, and it is rich in vitamins A, D, and E.

Tamanu Oil

Tamanu trees are native to Southeast Asia, where people believed that the tree was a sacred gift of nature and that a god hid in its branches. Tamanu oil is anti-aging and can be used to treat age spots and stretch marks.

Oil
for Hair

For

All hair types

Recommended Use

Once a week, or as often as you shampoo your hair

2 to 3 tablespoons coconut or sesame oil (depending on the length of your hair)

When I first heard that Indian women traditionally conditioned their hair before washing it to protect it from the drying effects of shampoo, it made complete sense to me. A lot of conventional shampoos can do more harm than good, with ingredients like sodium lauryl sulfates that strip the hair of its natural oils, which conventional conditioners do a poor job of replenishing. Oiling your hair is a simple practice that can help restore necessary moisture and bring lustrous shine back to your locks. It can be done weekly or monthly, as often as you need a deep conditioning, and you can continue to use your daily hair conditioner.

Brush or comb your hair thoroughly. Put the oil in a glass bowl. Heat a few inches of water in a saucepan and place the bowl in the water for a few minutes, until the oil is warm. Starting with the crown of your head and working downward and outward with your fingertips, massage the oil into the scalp by pinching and releasing with your fingertips. Rub the oil through the strands of hair, concentrating on the ends and adding more oil if needed. Leave on for 30 minutes, then wash your hair. For deep conditioning, you can leave the oil on overnight and wash it out in the morning.

To Combat Dandruff: Add a few drops of rose, lavender, geranium, or rosemary essential oil to your coconut or sesame oil, and really concentrate on spreading the oil on your scalp.

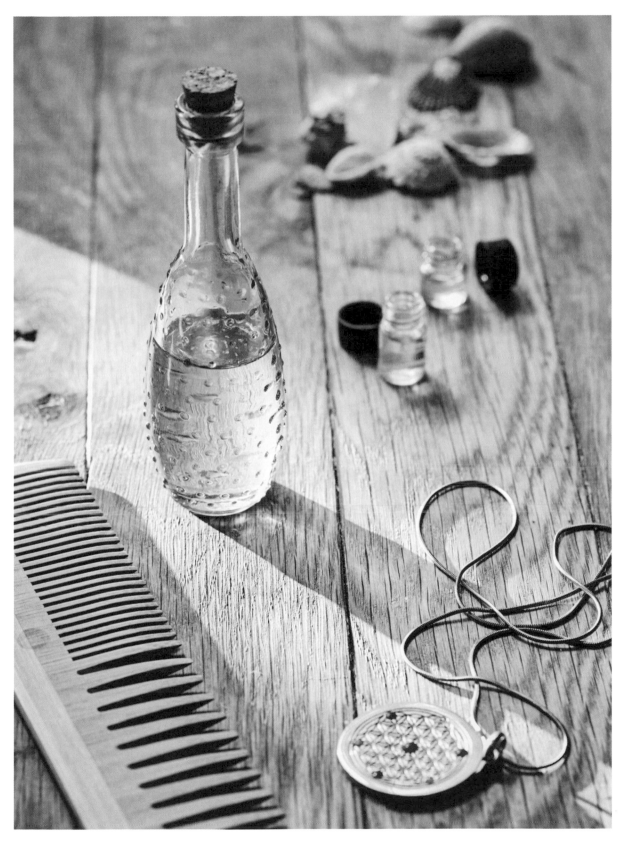

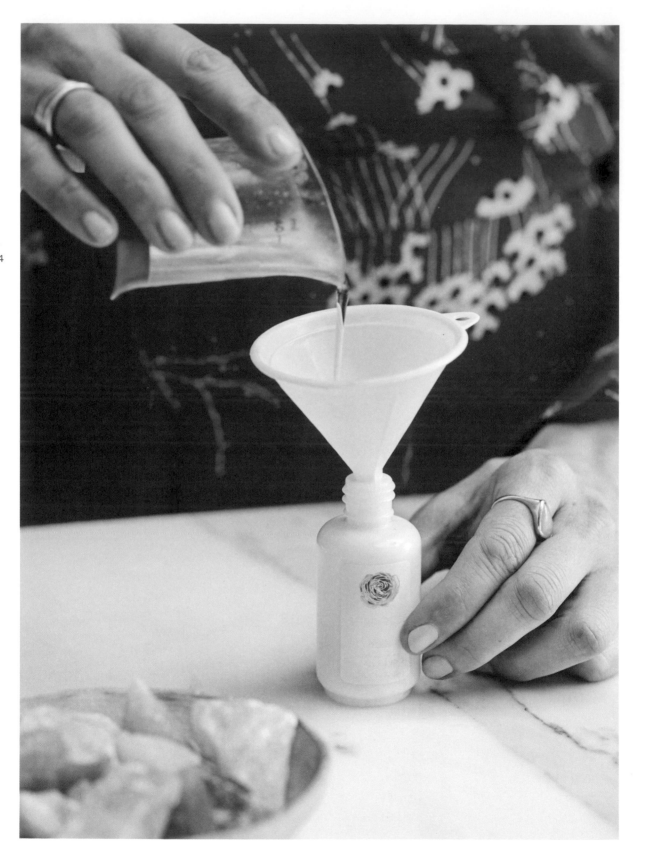

Nourishing
Face Oil

For
Normal to dry skin

Recommended Use
Twice a day, or as needed

2 tablespoons jojoba oil
1 tablespoon kukui nut oil
1 tablespoon rose hip oil
1 tablespoon argan oil
1 teaspoon sea buckthorn oil
A few drops of vitamin E oil
A few drops of an essential oil
   that you like

4-ounce glass bottle with cap
   or stopper

My face oil is my signature product. The idea to create it came to me during a Kundalini meditation, and I made it for myself and to give to my friends before I ever began making it to sell. It is wonderfully nourishing, it is anti-aging, and it feeds and comforts the skin. The oil is inspired by the Hindu goddesses Lalita, the one who dwells in a forest of bliss and wanders free; Parvati, the daughter of a mountain who is moved by love; and Lakshmi, who offers the most lasting forms of wealth, integrity, empathy, compassion, and love.

When I'm making the oil, I evoke the goddesses' blessings by playing mantras and imagining their presence with me in the studio. I make my face oil with rose to open the heart chakra, but you can customize yours with your favorite fragrance.

Mix the oils and transfer to the glass bottle. Use a few drops to moisturize your skin in the morning, at night, or whenever it needs to be replenished.

Shimmering
Body Oil

For
All skin types

Recommended Use
Use after bathing or before an
evening out

2 teaspoons mica, either gold
    or bronze
1 tablespoon shea butter or
    coconut oil
3 ounces sunflower seed oil
5 drops of vanilla essential oil
    (or any essential oil you prefer)

4-ounce glass bottle with stopper

This oil absolutely makes you glow! It's indulgent
and fun, and it smells heavenly. Mica is a natural
mineral dust that adds a hint of glimmer, making
this body oil perfect for a date night or when you're
wearing a beautiful dress and want to highlight
your skin.

Using a funnel, pour the mica into the glass bottle.
In a saucepan over low heat, melt the shea butter
or coconut oil, then add to the bottle. Pour in the
sunflower seed oil and the vanilla essential oil,
place the stopper in the bottle, and shake. Use
your fingertips to apply lovingly to your shoulders,
chest, and limbs.

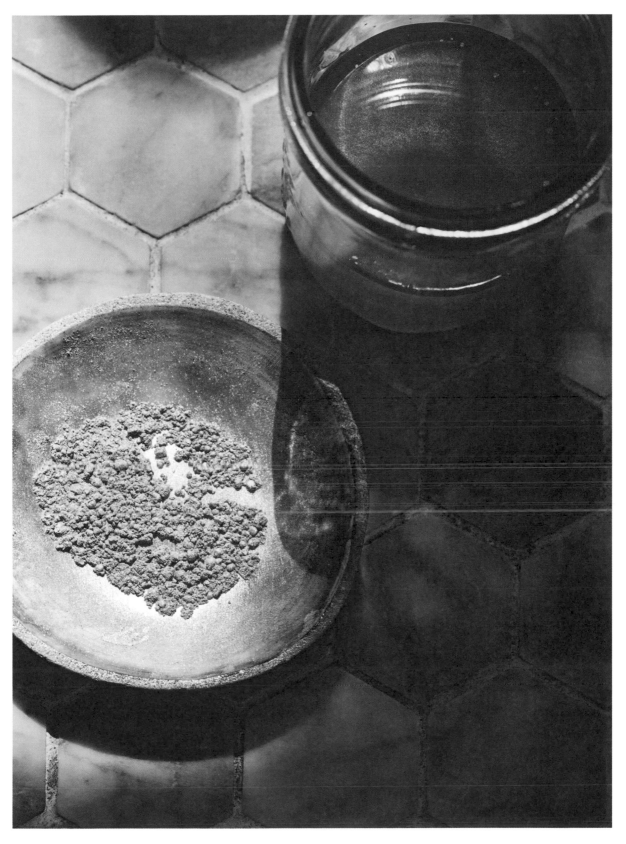

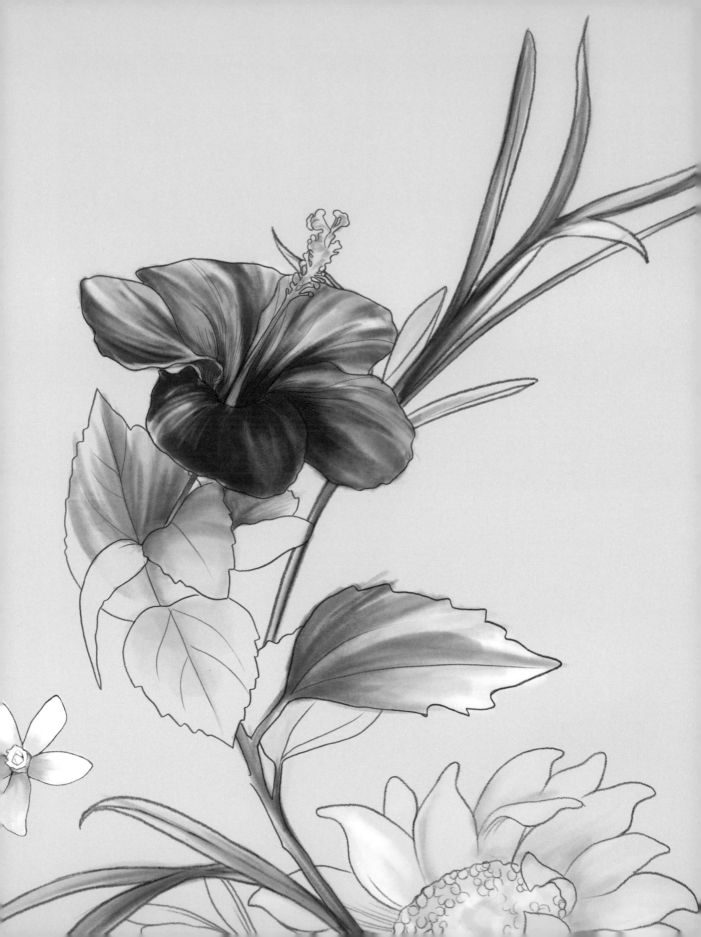

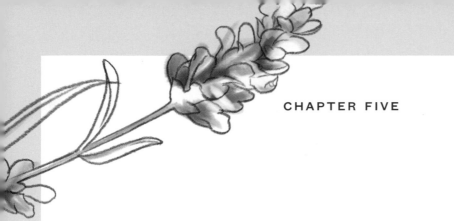
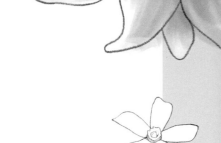

CHAPTER FIVE

Herbs, Tonics & Beauty Foods

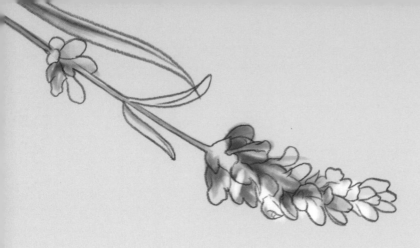

I don't know what else could be more worth it or more beneficial than putting extra effort into what you put into your body. Health is the true baseline of beauty, and no amount of bronzer can fake a radiant glow—the kind that extends past your cheeks to your eyes, smile, and entire being.

When I decided to change my life after my divorce, I started with food. I began growing some of my own vegetables, and I got chickens and honeybees. I had always shopped at the Santa Monica Farmers Market, and I rededicated myself to eating organic food and developing a relationship with the people who grew it.

I learned to eat to balance my hormones and nourish my body with healthy fats. A product of the nineties, I had been taught that fat was the worst thing to consume, so I avoided it at all costs. This left me depleted, anxious, and depressed, with dull skin and brittle hair. When I began to add healthy fats—like those found in avocado, coconut oil, and ghee—back into my diet, my body sighed with gratitude. I was finally replenishing my ojas.

However, we live in a world where it is impossible to always eat what benefits us, and that's where herbs and tonics come in. A few years ago, I started supplementing my diet with tonics, and I truly felt a change in my energy levels. I began

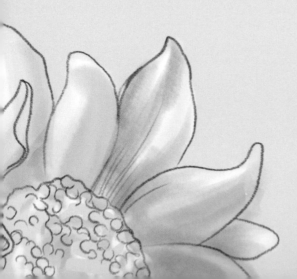

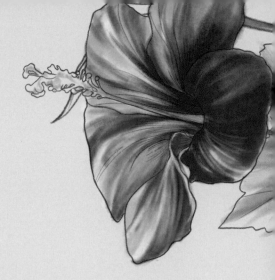

with ashwagandha and reishi, and now I take about four different tonics each day depending on the season and how I am feeling. I rarely drink coffee or alcohol. Tonics are what help me get up early, fight a midafternoon slump, or calm down before bed after a stressful day.

I also drink herbal teas to help beautify and flush out my system. Incorporating herbs into my wellness practice has helped strengthen my relationship with plants and nature. I grow my own chamomile and nettle, and I forage for herbs when I am on a hike or out for a walk. Even if you live in an apartment and can grow herbs only in a window box, your connection to the plant will be so much stronger if you have grown and harvested it yourself. You will feel so much more nourished.

The process of working with plants is incredibly intuitive, so rather than follow specific measurements and portion everything out with cups and spoons, I like to use my hands and see what feels good. I listen to my body to see what

it desires, and if I am making tea, I save the herbs to use in a mask, or I throw them into the garden so that I can funnel the energy into my being and back into the earth. Since the benefits of these herbs and spices will go directly into your bloodstream, always buy organic and source from the purest places possible.

Again, these herbs and other tonic ingredients are not regulated. Be certain to source them from reputable companies such as Dragon Herbs and Sun Potion (see Resources). You should experiment on your own to make sure you don't have allergies. For many people, tonics are new terrain, which is exciting, but you should exercise just as much caution as you would when taking a new vitamin or supplement.

Many of the following recipes were inspired by working with Nitsa Citrine of Sun Potion. Keep in mind that they are starting points to fuel your creativity and intuition. They are yours to play with and adapt.

My Favorite Beauty Foods

It's pretty amazing that the best thing you can do for your skin is to eat some of the delicious foods that come from Mama Earth. It's that easy! These are my go-to ingredients that I try to incorporate into my diet as much as I can, whether that means adding them to salads or grain bowls, using them as substitutes for less-healthy options, or snacking on them throughout the day. True beauty is about nourishment, not denial, and these foods will help you have lustrous hair, glowing skin, and juicy ojas.

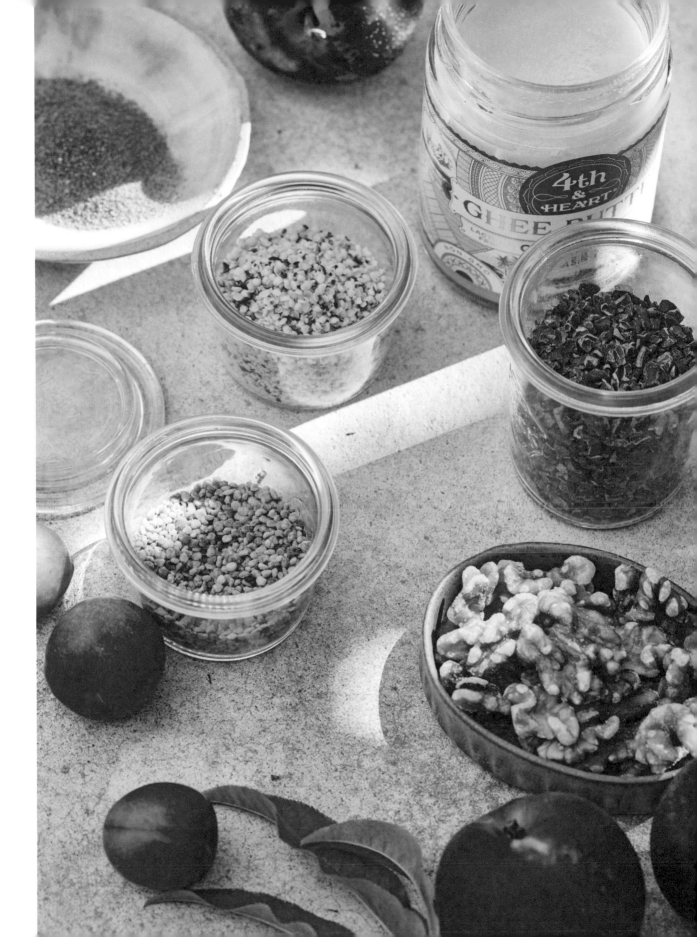

Almonds

I snack on almonds throughout the day, and soaking them first makes them easier to digest. They are full of vitamin E and biotin—which help repair brittle hair and nails and prevent dandruff—and copper, which aids in the production of elastin. (You know, that stuff that prevents wrinkles!)

Aloe Juice

Aloe juice is great for soothing dry skin and helps fight aging by keeping skin hydrated and firm. It also aids in digestion.

Avocados

I feel so lucky to live in California, where you can find avocados at every farmers' market, or even sometimes on the sidewalk! Avocados contain carotenoids, like alpha- and beta-carotene, which are what the skin needs to feel toned and dense. Avocados' monounsaturated fats help skin maintain moisture, and their vitamins E and C help prevent free-radical damage.

Bone Broth

I have a deep love for animals, and for most of my life I honored this by being a vegetarian. Eventually, I learned that I was deficient in certain vitamins and nutrients you can get only from animal protein, and now I supplement my diet with bone broth. In addition to providing necessary amino acids, it also has collagen and gelatin, both of which support healthy hair and skin.

Cacao Nibs

Cacao nibs are full of flavonoids, a kind of antioxidant that gives flower petals their pigment, helps create collagen, and also improves skin conditions like eczema. Cacao has forty times the antioxidants of blueberries, and it is also one of the best plant-based sources of iron and magnesium.

Chia Seeds

Chia is full of protein and mineral-dense nutrients, and it's high in fiber and omega-3 fatty acids. The seeds can keep you feeling full for some time and help with weight loss while providing a needed dose of healthy fat.

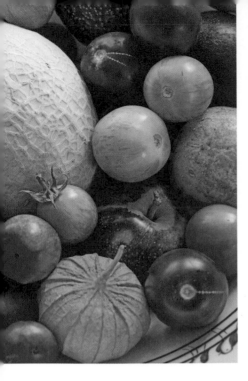
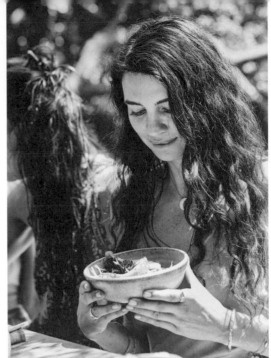

Coconut

I love everything coconut: coconut water, coconut oil, coconut meat, and coconut milk. Coconut water is an excellent source of calcium and electrolytes to help the skin and hair. Coconut oil is high in lauric acid, which fights inflammation and makes hair and skin strong and supple. In addition to being delicious, coconut meat is full of beneficial live enzymes and skin-beautifying minerals like magnesium, potassium, and copper. Coconut milk is creamy like dairy and rich in all sorts of fatty acids and lauric acids, which are really good for the skin, hair, and bones. It is also full of electrolytes.

Dates

In India and many parts of the Middle East, dates are a staple food that almost everyone consumes. They are not as popular in the West, but they should be! Dates are rich in vitamin B_6, which helps repair damaged cells and keep hair healthy. They are also a good source of antioxidants.

Ghee

Ghee, or traditional Ayurvedic clarified butter, keeps you supple and juicy, and it might be my number one beauty food. It is rich in vitamins A, E, and K, which are beneficial for hair, nails, skin, and joints. It increases digestive fire, improves the absorption of nutrients into the body, is nourishing to the ojas, and strengthens the nervous system and the brain. Ghee contains conjugated linolenic acid, which inhibits the growth of cancer cells and is a source of good cholesterol. Traditionally used in Ayurvedic medicine as a topical cure for blisters and burns, ghee may also help in minimizing stomach acid while simultaneously repairing the gut's lining. I like to take a spoonful of ghee every morning, or you can use it in place of cooking oil in most recipes.

Hemp Seeds

Hemp seeds are superseeds, high in essential fatty acids, vitamin E and B vitamins, and easily digestible protein. They are perfect as a topping for breakfast oats or in a smoothie.

Juicy Fruits

Think peaches, mangoes, papayas, and watermelon. When fruits are ripe, they can turn into *rasa*, or "nutritional fluid," which enhances the ojas. You are nourishing your body with all of the juicy moisture and nutrients and your spirit with the bright colors and sweet flavors.

Oil

Just as many of us have been taught to avoid using oil on our skin, we've also been taught to avoid oil in our cooking and are missing out on necessary healthy fats because of it. There are so many wonderful oils that you can use to cook with, dress salads, or add to smoothies. Some of my favorites are almond, sesame, coconut, olive, hemp, and flaxseed. Experiment with different ones for different uses, and find what best suits your palate and your body.

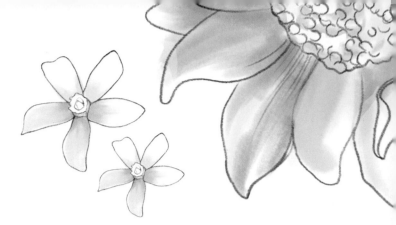

Raisins

Raisins contain resveratrol, which is a powerful polyphenol that helps protect against aging and free-radical damage, in addition to cancer and heart disease. Polyphenols are also rich in vitamins A and E, which help support the production of new skin cells.

Sesame Seeds

Sesame seeds are one of the oldest foods known to man. They are incredibly rich in minerals like selenium (which prevents UV damage, hyperpigmentation, and inflammation) and magnesium, high in protein and amino acids, and rich in zinc, which can help prevent acne. I also love to use tahini (a paste made from sesame seeds) in salad dressings and dips.

Sunflower Seeds

Sunflower seeds are a good source of protein and are rich in amino acids like tryptophan, which give them a calming effect. The vitamin E, high folic acid count, zinc, and B vitamins sunflower seeds contain provide a big boost for hormones, and a handful of sunflower seeds every day can increase testosterone in men and support their sperm count.

Sweet Potato

Sweet potatoes are rich in vitamins C and D, which help produce collagen to keep skin youthful and elastic.

Whole Grains

Processed grains can cause your insulin levels to spike, which results in acne and other inflammatory skin problems. Whole grains don't do this, and they are also rich in selenium. I like quinoa, forbidden rice, and gluten-free oats.

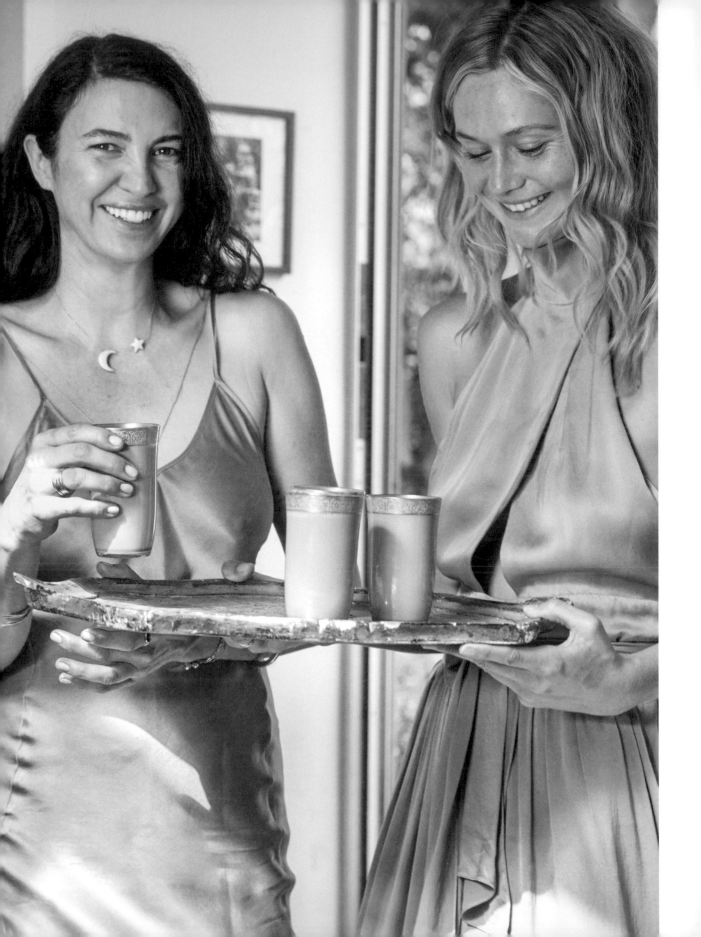

My Favorite Herbs & Tonics

Tonics draw upon Chinese medicine and Ayurvedic traditions. Used in small doses, they tone the system over time. You won't feel a jolt, like you do from caffeine, but instead you'll notice subtle changes in your energy levels that leave you feeling more restored, balanced, and invigorated. Tonics typically come in powder or tincture form, and you can simply mix them in water and sip them straight. However, since many have a bitter or very earthy taste, I often incorporate them into hot beverages or smoothies.

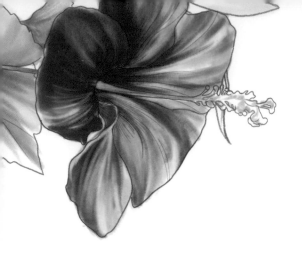

These tonic ingredients have not been evaluated by the FDA, and you should experiment by taking a tablespoon of each in water to see if you have an adverse reaction. If you are particularly worried about taking a tonic, check with your physician, as you would before taking any new vitamins or supplements. Following are some of the herbs that I like to have on hand to create my tonics.

Amalaki Fruit

Amalaki fruit (also called Indian gooseberry) is known as "the fruit of immortality," and it works on the bowels and digestive system, which are important for clearing the skin. In addition to being very rich in vitamin C, it supports the inner lining of the digestive tract, can help slow aging and reverse sun damage, and protects the liver.

Ashitaba

A powerful tonic from a leafy green Japanese plant that is known for its regenerative powers and ability to heal itself, ashitaba promotes glowing skin and good digestion. It is high in B vitamins (one of the only plants that provides vitamin B_{12}) and vitamin C, and it helps eliminate toxins. It can also help with weight reduction.

Ashwagandha

In Sanskrit, *ashwagandha* means "smell of a horse," because it is supposed to impart the vigor and stamina of a stallion. Ashwagandha comes from the crushed leaves and roots of the winter cherry tree. It is an adaptogen, which means it works by adapting to your body's needs to reduce stress or provide more energy. In Ayurveda, it was traditionally prescribed to help people recover from illness. It is an anti-inflammatory and can prevent anxiety and depression.

Astragalus

Astragalus is a root that helps to lower cortisol and strengthen the immune system to fight disease. It has long been used in Chinese medicine as an adaptogen.

Chaga

Chaga is a mushroom found on the trunks of birch trees, and it is known as the "king healer mushroom" in Chinese medicine. It is rich in zinc and B vitamins, and it is a powerful adaptogen that aids in immune response and provides energy.

Chyawanprash

Chyawanprash is an ancient Ayurvedic blend of thirty-five ingredients (herbs, spices, and fruits) taken as a supplement for wellness, rejuvenation, and longevity. Made with amalaki fruit, sesame, and honey, it tastes like jam. Chyawanprash aids in eliminating toxins, boosting the immune system, and strengthening the organs, in addition to lifting the libido and balancing hormones. Its antioxidants are good for skin and hair, and it is good for balancing all the doshas.

Cistanche

Cistanche is a desert plant that has been used in Chinese medicine for thousands of years; Genghis Khan reportedly consumed it every day. It is known to be a mood-supporting herb, helps detoxify the kidneys, and enhances sexual power for both men and women. Some species of cistanche are endangered, so make sure you buy yours from a reputable source.

Cordyceps

Chinese medicine has long used this fungus to shrink cancerous tumors, and it is also known to increase endurance and performance.

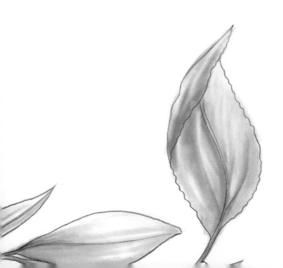

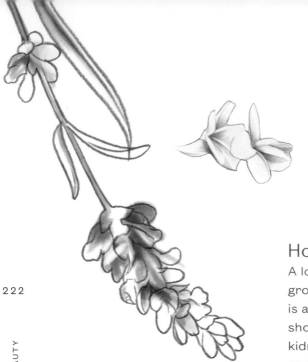

Ho Shou Wu

A longevity tonic made from the root of a plant that grows in China's mountainous regions, ho shou wu is also great for growing thick, lustrous hair. Ho shou wu provides a boost to the endocrine system, kidneys, and liver, which improves energy, stamina, and immunity. (Some people have had adverse reactions to ho shou wu, however, so check with your doctor if you have any concerns.)

Maca

Maca is the superfood adaptogen cousin of broccoli and cabbage. It grows high in the mountains of Peru and helps elevate endorphins to make people feel more alive. It increases stamina, provides energy, balances hormones in both men and women, and can help increase focus. It's loaded with amino acids and essential minerals.

Mucuna Pruriens

Sometimes called kapikachhu, mucuna pruriens is a legume grown in Asia and Africa and is known as the "dopamine" bean, because it can increase the levels of dopamine in the brain. It's excellent for combating mood swings, depression, and addiction. It stimulates the pituitary gland to regulate hormonal imbalances and can promote fertility in both men and women.

Pearl Powder

This is one of my favorite ingredients for luminous beauty and lustrous hair. Taking pearl powder internally can boost collagen and give the body more calcium and trace minerals.

Pine Pollen

Pine pollen has been an aphrodisiac and longevity food in ancient cultures for centuries. This adaptogen has twenty amino acids, including eight essential ones. I love the golden hue of the powder and can feel its vitality working on me right away.

Reishi

Reishi is known as the "queen healer mushroom," and in Chinese medicine, it is tied to success, well-being, and longevity. It is a powerful adaptogen that is anti-inflammatory, antioxidant, cancer fighting, and stress reducing. It also helps to lower blood pressure and cholesterol.

Shatavari

Sometimes known as wild asparagus, shatavari is an Ayurvedic herb. It balances hormones, soothes digestion, and promotes immunity. It helps to reduce acidity in the body and balance pH. It can help regulate the menstrual cycle and also promote thick, healthy hair.

Tocos

Tocos is soluble rice bran that is full of vitamin E, which is important for healthy skin and connective tissue. Its creamy vanilla taste makes it a wonderful addition to smoothies or tonics.

Triphala

Triphala means "three fruits," and it is made from amalaki, which manages Pitta and supports the liver and the immune system; bibhitaki, which is good for Kapha and supports the respiratory system; and haritaki, which removes toxins and is good for all three doshas.

All of these recipes make one serving but can easily be doubled or tripled for sharing. Some simple kitchen items, like a blender, cheesecloth, and a saucepan, are required.

Rejuvenating Tonic

1 tablespoon ashwagandha
1 tablespoon mucuna pruriens
1 teaspoon raw honey
1 to 2 cups hot water (according
    to taste)
Almond milk

This tonic is excellent for balancing the nervous system and doshas. I take it when I need to lift my spirits, even out my moods, and feel my vitality.

In a cup, mix the ashwagandha, mucuna pruriens, and honey in the hot water. Place some almond milk in a blender and blend on high speed until frothy, then scoop out the foam to top the drink. (Save the remaining liquid for another use.)

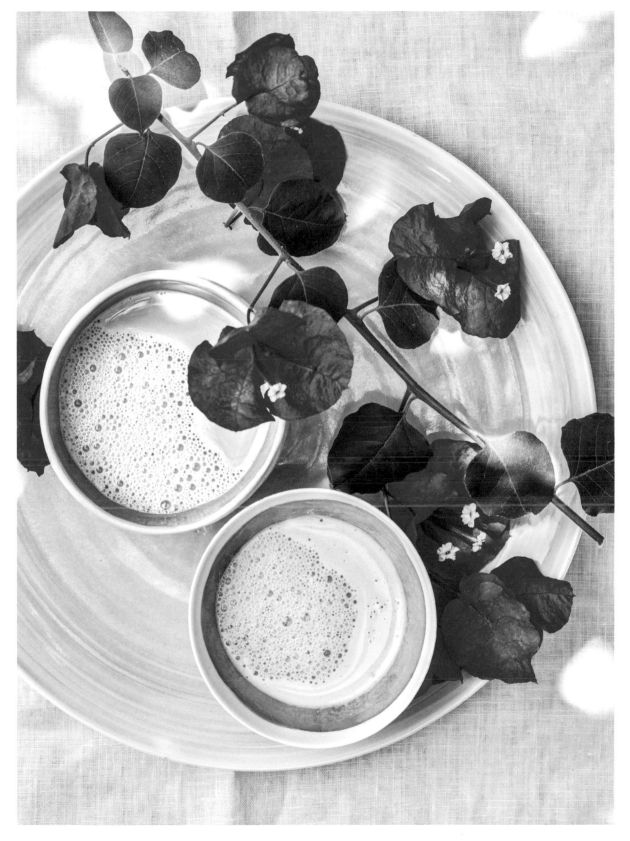

Restful Radiance Tonic

1 cup milk, preferably raw
  (see page 147)
1 teaspoon ghee
1 teaspoon shatavari
1 teaspoon raw honey

This tonic is wonderful after a long day, and it will help send you off into your beauty sleep. It also helps balance Vata and Pitta issues, and the ghee nourishes ojas with healthy fat.

Warm the milk in a saucepan. Add the ghee, shatavari, and honey and stir until the ghee and honey have dissolved. Pour into a cup.

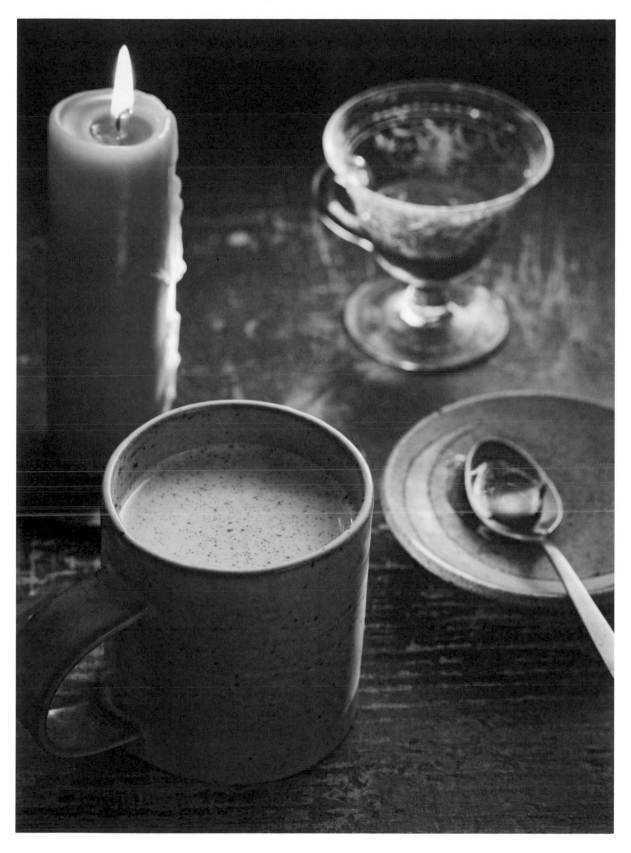

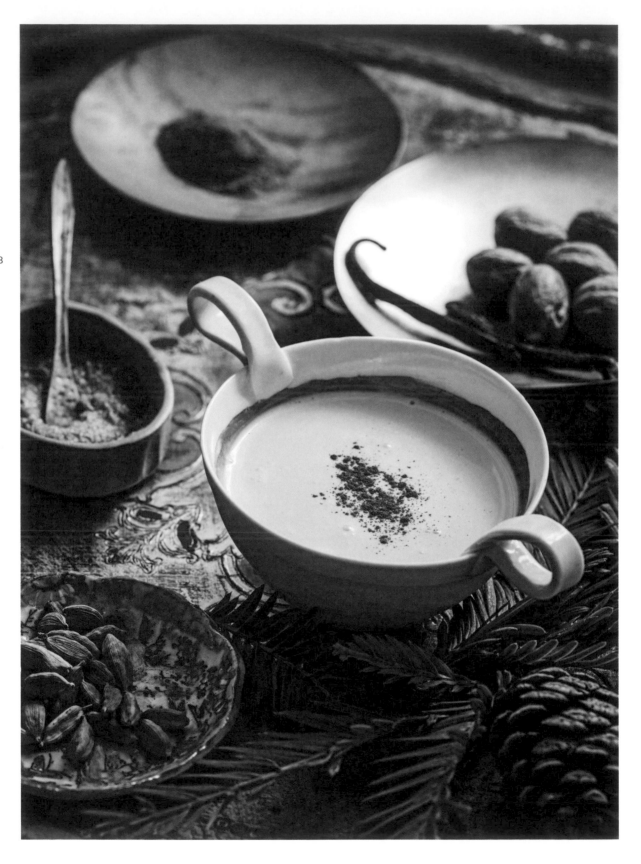

Celestial Nog

Pumpkin Seed Milk

1 cup raw sprouted
   pumpkin seeds
1 teaspoon organic vanilla extract
1 teaspoon maple syrup

1 cup coconut cream
3 Medjool dates, soaked (optional)
1 tablespoon tocos
1 teaspoon pine pollen
½ teaspoon ho shou wu
½ teaspoon mucuna pruriens
½ teaspoon astragalus
1 teaspoon freshly ground nutmeg
⅛ teaspoon freshly ground cardamom
⅛ teaspoon ground cinnamon
⅛ teaspoon ground cloves
⅛ teaspoon turmeric
⅛ teaspoon sea salt

The holidays are a time to bask in the golden light of love and abundance, and I adore everything about Christmas—including eggnog. However, traditional eggnog is full of sugar and dairy, and I am sensitive to both. A few seasons ago, my friend Nitsa Citrine, of Sun Potion, and I created this holiday treat that captures the yuletide flavor and leaves us feeling healthy, vibrant, and joyful. In addition to being delicious, it will give your immune system a much-needed boost during a stressful, busy time of year.

Make the pumpkin seed milk: In a bowl, soak the pumpkin seeds in water to cover overnight in the refrigerator (if left at room temperature, it can mold). In the morning, strain out the seeds, put them in a blender, and blend them with 2 cups water. Strain the liquid through cheesecloth, discarding the solids. Put the liquid back in the blender and blend with the vanilla and maple syrup.

Warm the pumpkin seed milk in a saucepan, taking care not to bring it to a full boil to preserve living enzymes. Remove from the heat. Add the coconut cream, dates (if using), herbs, spices, and salt. Put the mixture in the blender and pulse for about a minute on high speed. Pour into a cup, and for a beautiful touch, garnish with a final pinch of spice.

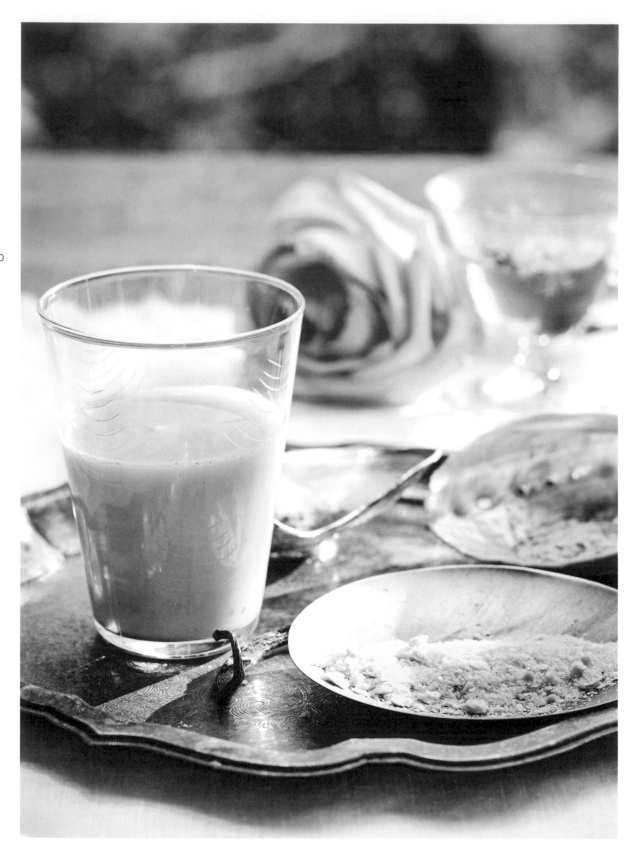

Libido-Enhancing Tonic

1 cup hot water
¼ cup almond milk
1 teaspoon pine pollen
1 teaspoon ho shou wu
1 teaspoon ashwagandha
1 teaspoon cistanche
1 teaspoon maca
¼ teaspoon vanilla powder
¼ cup tocos
Raw honey to taste
Turmeric, for sprinkling

This tonic is great for both men and women. In addition to waking up your libido, it also beautifies your hair. This is my daily happy-hour drink to combat my four o'clock slump.

In a bowl, stir together the hot water and almond milk, then add the herbs, vanilla, and tocos. Add honey to your desired sweetness, then transfer the mixture to a blender and pulse a few times so it gets nice and frothy. Pour into a drinking glass, and finish with a sprinkle of turmeric on top.

Summer
Lover Tonic

12 ounces jun or kombucha
2 teaspoons pine pollen
1 teaspoon mucuna pruriens
A squeeze of lemon juice
Raspberries, for garnish
Strawberries, for garnish
Mint leaves, for garnish

In addition to being a wonderful aphrodisiac, pine pollen contributes to immune health, balanced hormones, and firm, clear skin. I like to mix it with jun, a bubbly fermented drink made from green tea and honey, or kombucha to make this refreshing pick-me-up.

Pour the jun or kombucha into a drinking glass, add the pine pollen and mucuna pruriens, and stir until mixed well. Add the lemon juice, then garnish with berries and mint leaves.

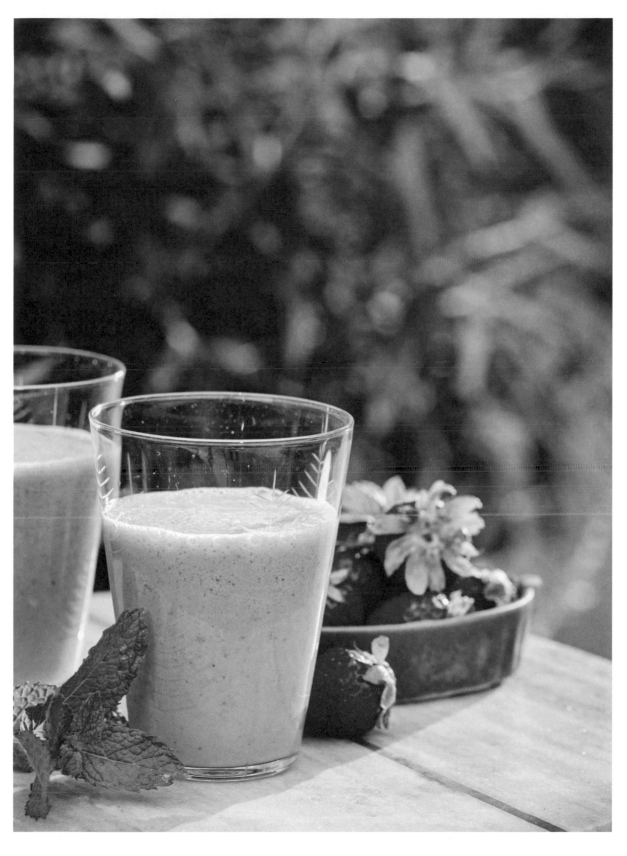

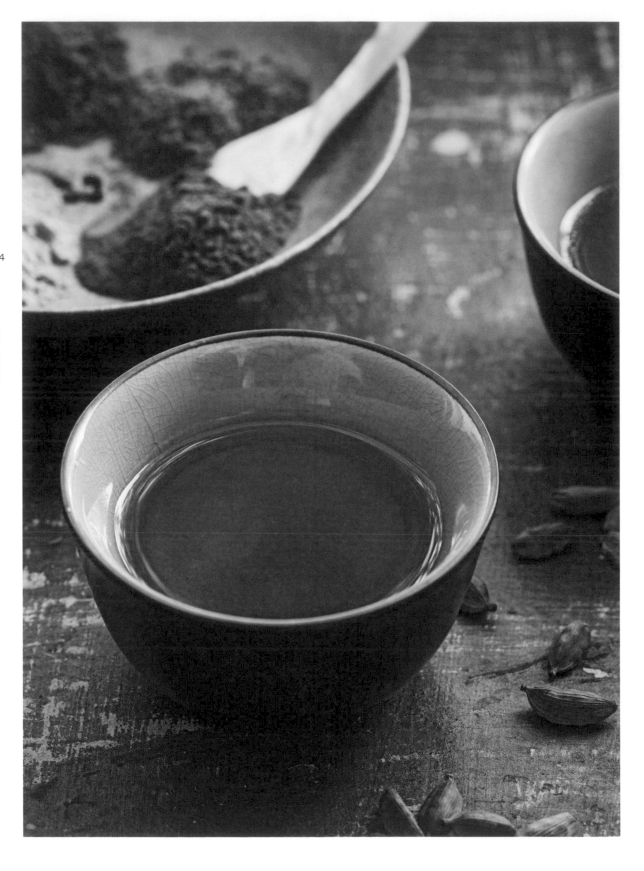

Immune-Boosting Tonic

1 gynostemma tea bag
1 cup hot water
1 teaspoon reishi
1 teaspoon chaga
1 teaspoon cordyceps
Coconut sugar or raw honey to
    taste (optional)
Coconut milk to taste (optional)
Cardamom, for sprinkling
Cinnamon, for sprinkling

Gynostemma is a balancing herb that encourages reflection and self-awareness. It naturally calms the digestive tract and lowers blood pressure. As an adaptogen, it responds to what your body needs, so it is calming when you are overexcited and provides energy when you need stimulation. It can help you cope with trauma and fatigue, and you can drink as much as you like, as it is impossible to overdo it. I like to use it as a base for a wellness tonic that harnesses the power of mushrooms (a good way to protect yourself during cold and flu season). The mushrooms can have a very bitter taste, so I sweeten them with coconut milk, spices, and a little honey or coconut sugar.

In a bowl, steep the gynostemma in the hot water for 3 to 5 minutes. Transfer to a blender and combine with the reishi, chaga, and cordyceps. Add the sweetener and coconut milk (if using) and blend until frothy. Pour into a cup, and top with a sprinkle of cardamom and cinnamon.

Cacao Maca
Cloud Smoothie

2 cups almond milk
1 banana
1 tablespoon chia seeds
1 tablespoon maca
1 tablespoon cacao
1 tablespoon organic vanilla extract
1 tablespoon coconut oil
Dash of cinnamon
Raw honey to taste
4 ice cubes
Crushed cacao nibs, for garnish
    (optional)

I love chocolate, and smoothies are an addiction in my house; this recipe combines both. I always joke that it should come with a warning, because maca can really elevate the libido. I know a lady whose husband is very pleased when she makes maca smoothies! The banana makes this one filling and full of potassium and magnesium, and the chia seeds are a good source of omega-3 fatty acids. Maca is always a pick-me-up, so I'll often make this smoothie to get me going in the morning, or when my adrenals need an extra boost in the afternoon.

Put the almond milk, banana, chia seeds, maca, cacao, vanilla, coconut oil, cinnamon, honey, and ice in the blender, and blend for 2 minutes. Pour into a drinking glass, and if you like, top with crushed cacao nibs for extra crunchy goodness.

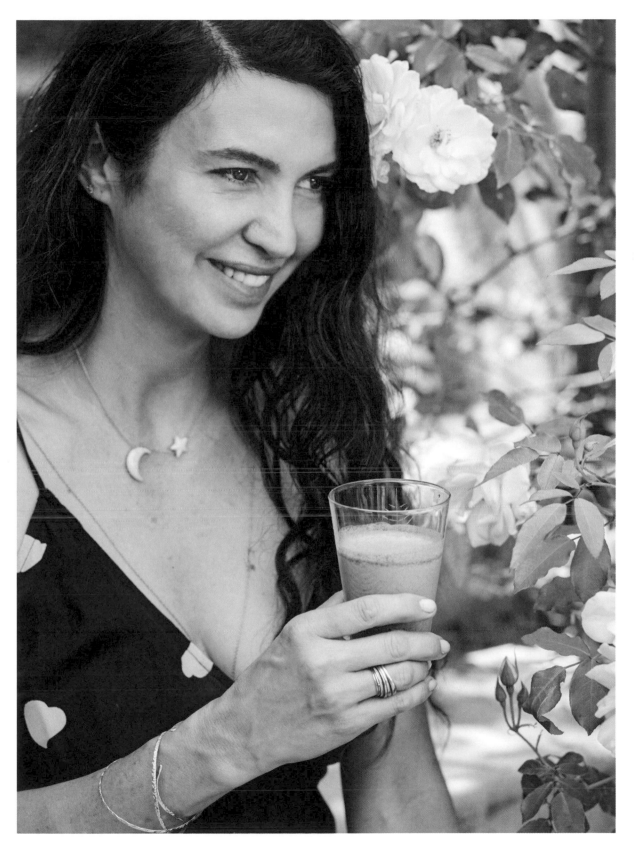

237

HERBS, TONICS & BEAUTY FOODS

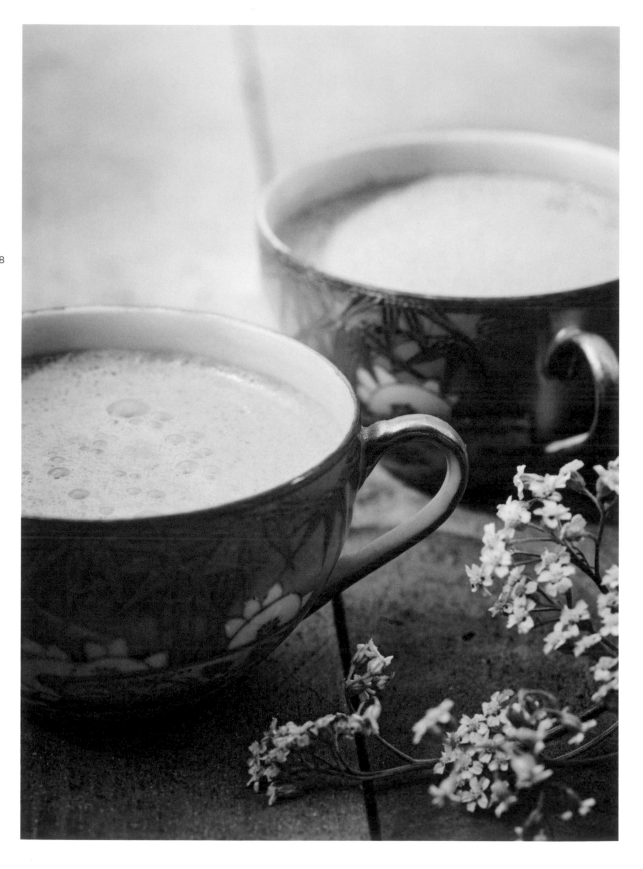

Magical Matcha

¾ cup almond milk
1 teaspoon matcha
¼ cup hot water
½ teaspoon pine pollen
½ teaspoon mucuna pruriens
1 teaspoon tocos

I love matcha for its sweet, grassy flavor and because it is rich in chlorophyll and antioxidants and boosts the metabolism while calming the mind. It also helps neutralize free radicals, which can help prevent premature aging. I like to make this latte in the morning.

Heat the almond milk in a saucepan. In a bowl or cup, whisk the matcha with the hot water until blended. Put both liquids in a blender with the pine pollen, mucuna pruriens, and tocos and blend until smooth. Pour into a cup.

Golden Milk

⅛ teaspoon turmeric

½ cup water

8 ounces milk, preferably raw
  (see page 147), or any kind of
  milk or nut milk that you like

2 tablespoons almond oil

Raw honey to taste

⅛ teaspoon cardamom or ghee
  (optional)

⅛ teaspoon ground black pepper
  (optional)

Golden milk is one of my favorite tonics. I often have it in the morning, or as a delicious after-dinner treat. I find it to be incredibly soothing and comforting, and a few years ago, in the middle of a very emotionally taxing time, Golden Milk was the only thing that consistently sounded good to me. It is full of anti-inflammatory turmeric, which aids stiff joints and improves brain function. Blending turmeric with a little black pepper enables the body to more easily absorb the turmeric, and the almond oil is a dose of healthy fat.

In a blender, combine the turmeric, water, milk, almond oil, and honey. Pulse until well blended, then strain the liquid through cheesecloth into a cup, discarding the solids. Drink warm or cool, topped with cardamom or ghee and pepper (if using).

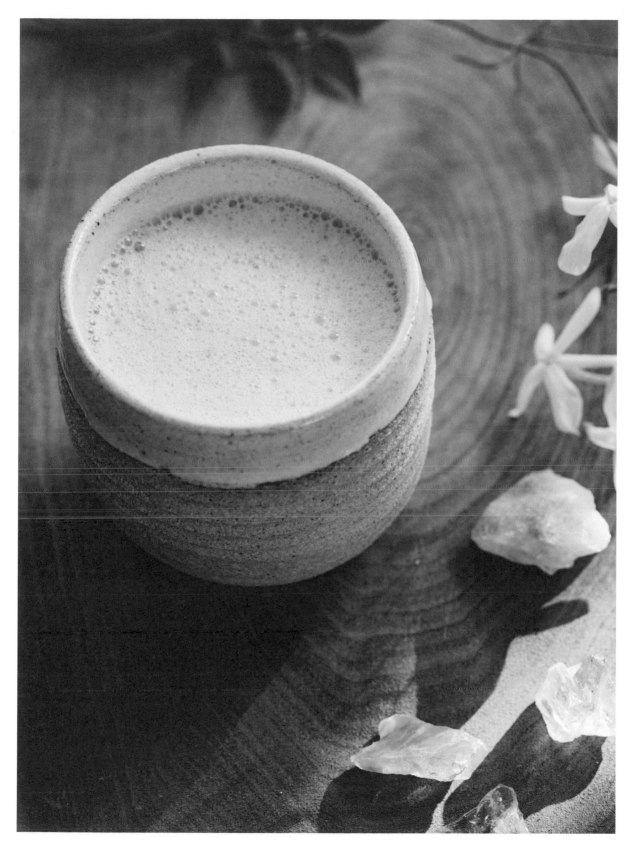

Herbal Teas & Spices

One way in which I can honor the earth and my body is by drinking herbal infusions or teas every day. I have so much respect for the properties of these wondrous plants. Many of the minerals and vitamins that lead to beautiful skin and hair, and balanced hormones, are derived from drinking them. I grow a lot of these herbs now—some that are even considered weeds!

Create a ritual out of brewing and drinking these teas by making a big jar of tea and setting it in the sun to absorb life-giving energy, or putting it outside at night to absorb the moon's calming influence. You can also just make a simple cup whenever you are thirsty! I sip these teas throughout the day, hot or cold depending on the season, and I am rarely without my giant mason jar of tea when I am at home.

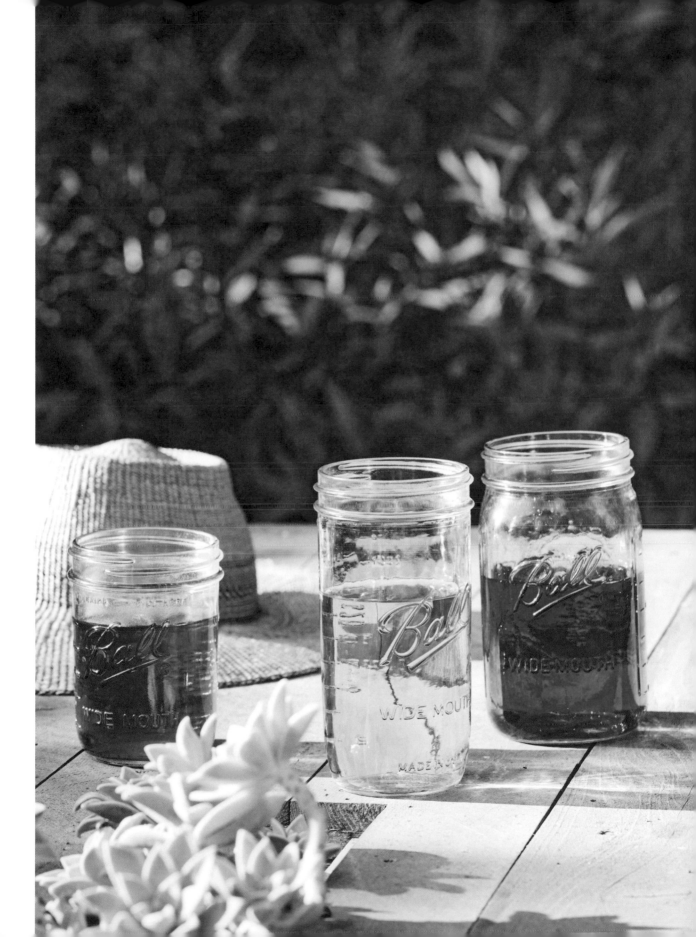

Daily
Detox Tea

¼ to ½ teaspoon dried whole
   coriander seeds
¼ to ½ teaspoon dried whole
   cumin seeds
¼ to ½ teaspoon dried fennel seeds
1 cup hot water

This traditional Ayurvedic tea lights digestive fires to restore vitality and eliminate sluggishness. Often just called digestive tea, it is mildly bitter, which helps promote clear skin by creating more bile in the liver. I like to drink this tea after meals, or just sip it throughout the day.

In a bowl, mix the coriander seeds, cumin seeds, and fennel seeds and steep in the hot water for 3 to 5 minutes. Strain the liquid through cheesecloth into a drinking glass and discard the solids. Drink warm or cool.

Note: You can adjust the amounts according to taste. It is a subtle tea, so I like mine a little bit stronger.

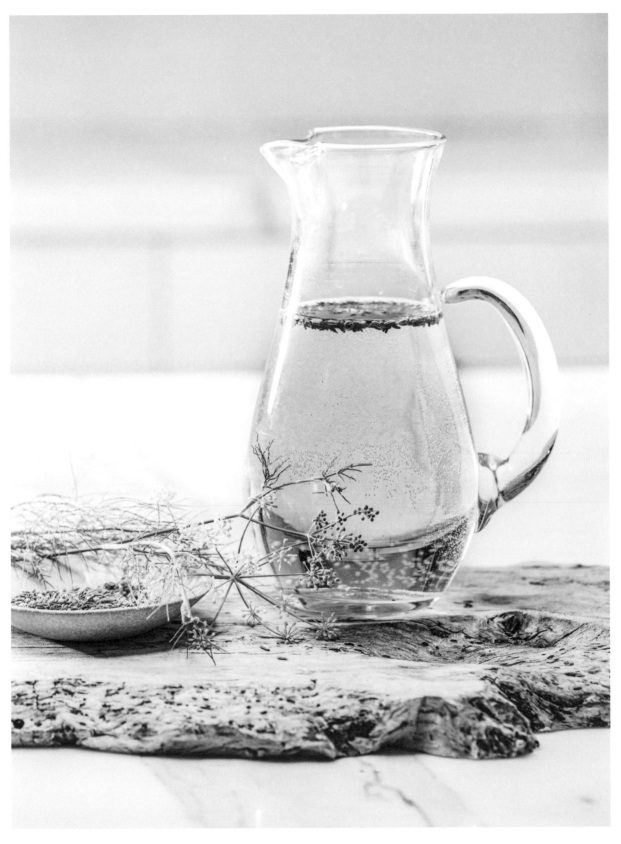

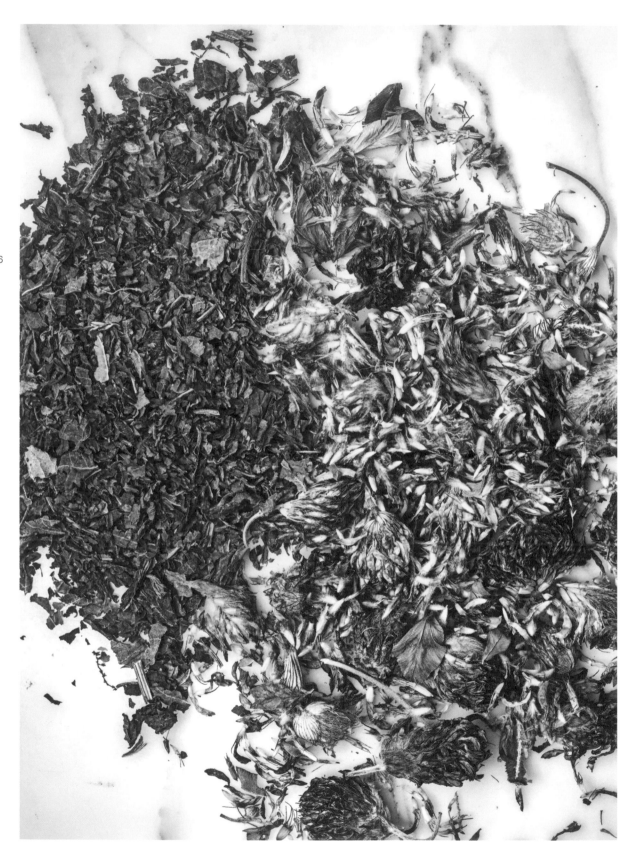

Nettle & Red Clover Tea

1 tablespoon dried red clover
   blossoms
1 tablespoon dried nettle
1 cup hot water

Nettle is one of the best plants you can get, as it is very nourishing for the adrenals. It is anti-inflammatory, helps combat hay fever, relieves dry skin conditions, and stimulates hair growth. Red clover reduces anxiety and depression, helps with PMS, and strengthens bones. There is something magical about watching the dried red clover blossoms bloom in hot water, and I think that is a wonderful metaphor for this tea: it will help you bloom.

Place the clover blossoms and nettle in a bowl with the hot water and allow to steep for 3 to 5 minutes. Strain the liquid through cheesecloth into a cup, discarding the solids, and drink warm or cool.

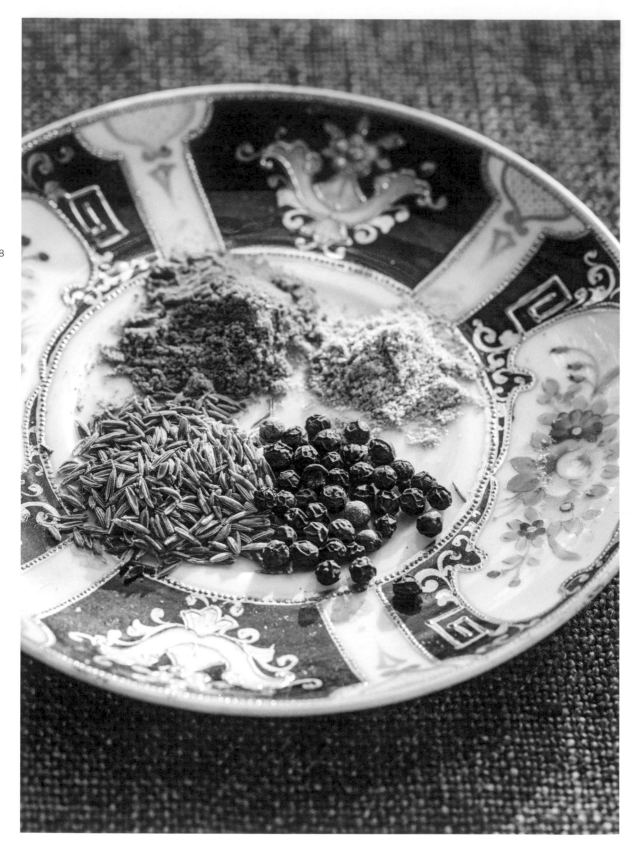

Skin-Nourishing Spice Mix

3 tablespoons turmeric
3 tablespoons ground coriander
4 tablespoons ground fennel seeds
(you can also sauté them for
flavor, and add them whole)
1 tablespoon ground black pepper

Glass jar with lid

This spice mix promotes digestion without heating up the body, helping to heal tissues, reduce inflammation, and calm skin issues. I like to sprinkle it on roasted vegetables, quinoa dishes, and salads for extra nourishment and flavor.

Mix the turmeric, coriander, fennel seeds, and black pepper in the glass jar. The mixture will keep for up to several months in your spice cabinet.

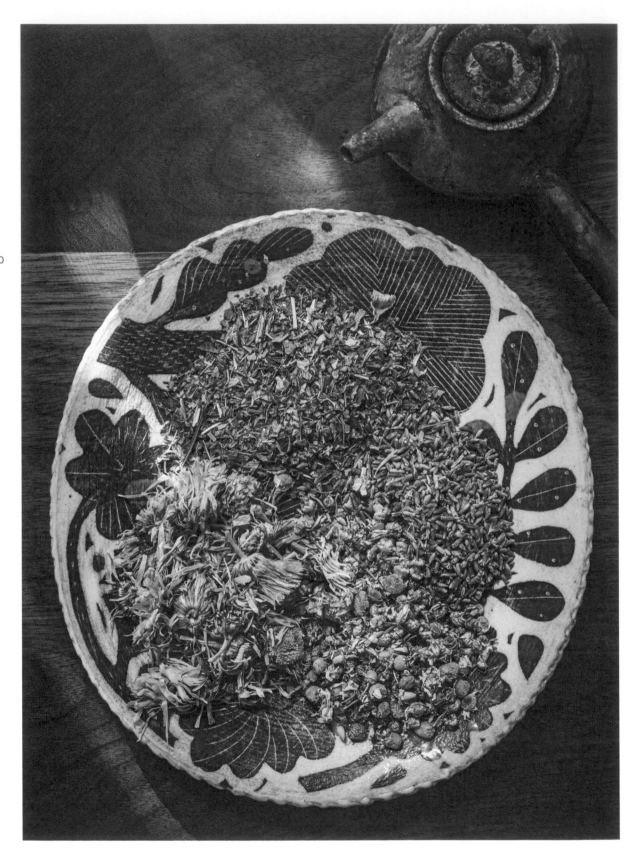

Bedtime Tea

1 tablespoon dried chamomile
1 tablespoon dried skullcap
1 tablespoon dried lavender
1 tablespoon dried calendula
2 cups hot water

This tea quiets your mind at the end of a busy day and will send you off to sleep feeling relaxed and refreshed. Skullcap soothes the nervous system, calendula and chamomile are both calming and anti-inflammatory, and lavender aids digestion and combats insomnia.

In a bowl, mix the chamomile, skullcap, lavender, calendula, and hot water and steep for 3 to 5 minutes. Strain the liquid through cheesecloth into a cup, discarding the solids. Drink warm or cool.

Note: Calendula and chamomile are both excellent for the skin when used externally as well. Lay the blossoms on your face while they are still warm, and cover with a cloth. The chamomile reduces dark circles and tightens skin, while calendula soothes breakouts and irritated or sunburned skin.

Skin
Ambrosia Tea

3 tablespoons dried red hibiscus
3 tablespoons dried calendula
1 cup hot water
Raw honey to taste (optional)

In Greek myths, ambrosia was only for the gods and goddesses, as it was thought to bring long life and immortality to anyone who consumed it. I call this mix of hibiscus and calendula "ambrosia for the skin" because it is rejuvenating and anti-aging. Hibiscus tea has always had a special place in my heart because the beautiful red flower is often given as an offering to the Hindu goddesses Lakshmi and Kali. As a tea, these red flowers are full of vitamin C and lightly detoxifying. A pitcher of this is a bright and colorful addition to any springtime table.

In a bowl, mix the hibiscus and calendula with the hot water and steep for an hour. As the mixture is cooling, add honey to taste (if using) and stir until blended. Strain the liquid through cheesecloth into a cup, discarding the solids. Drink hot, warm, or over ice.

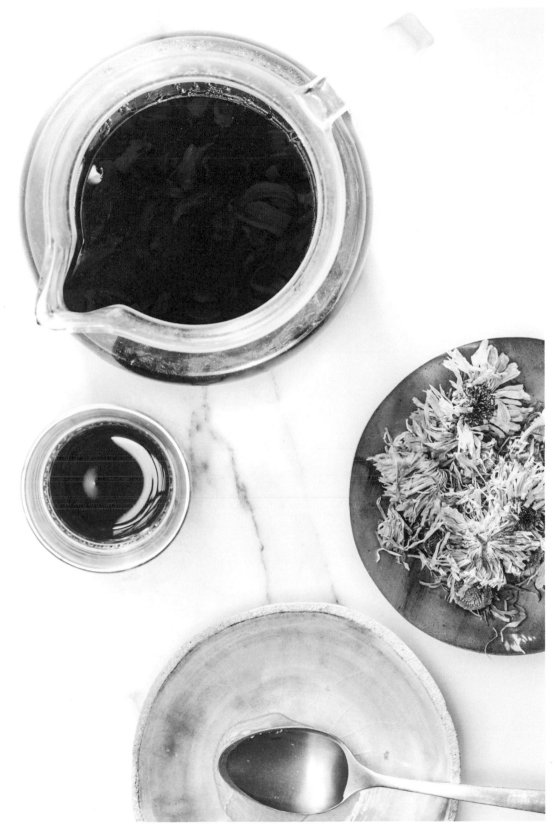

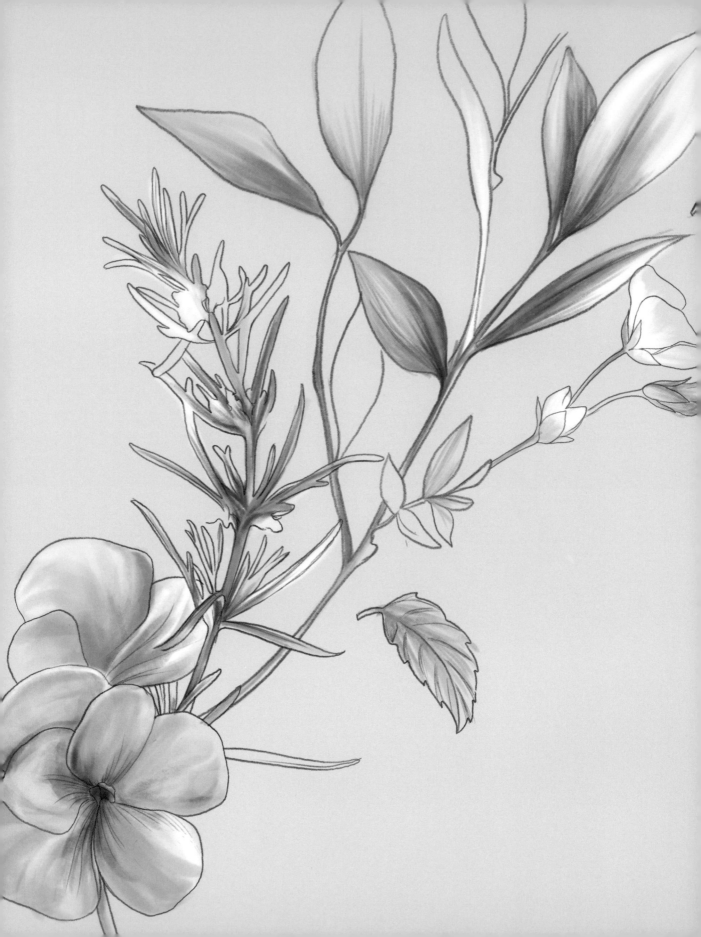

CHAPTER SIX

Essential Oils

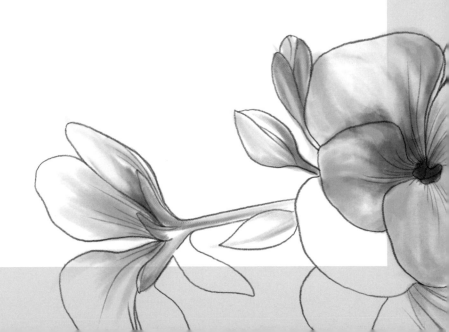

Our olfactory sense is intimately connected to our memories, and scents can transport and transform us. Even now, the fragrances of rose water and saffron take me instantly back to the bazaars of Iran, where I am a child trailing after my mother while she does her shopping.

One of the most heart-opening experiences of my adult life was going to see Amma, the hugging saint, for the first time.
It was a very unusual and beautiful experience, and I attribute that in part to the power of essential oils. Amma wears a combination of sandalwood and rose, and you can smell it before she even arrives. It's uncanny—almost like the fragrance of her aura enters the room before she does.

Amma's religion is love, and in her lifetime, she has hugged more than 34 million people. Often, you have to wait in line for hours to see her. In that time, you start to wonder, *Is this worth it? What is this? Will it work?* Then, when she embraces you, all of that goes away as you are enveloped in the scent of roses. Even though she has been sitting, without getting up to eat or go to the bathroom, for twelve hours, she is not fatigued, and she exudes this scent that is uplifting, divine, and comforting all at once. I am always moved to tears and overwhelmed with gratitude in her presence. I have gone to visit

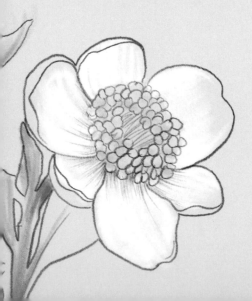

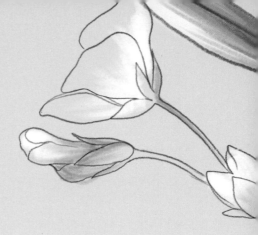

her many times, and each time, I feel like her scent stays in my nose for days after she has left.

Essential oils are a gift from the natural world. The name actually comes from the term *quintessential oils*, which is based on the idea that the fifth element (after fire, earth, air, and water) was ether, or "quintessence." People believed that these oils actually captured the spirit of the plant. Essential oils can be made from bark, leaves, petals, stems, and roots through processes like steam distillation, cold-pressing, and resin tapping (it all depends on the individual plant). As they are highly concentrated, a little goes a long way.

Essential oils have been used in healing for thousands of years, in cultures from Greek to Persian, Roman to Assyrian, and essential oil vessels have even been found in Egyptian tombs. Ancient priestesses would carry different resins or essential oils in pouches against their bodies for power and protection. Essential oils are a speedy remedy that helps us to heal just by removing a cap and breathing in. Different essential oils can help to improve mood, lower stress, reduce pain, quell nausea, banish headaches, balance hormones, induce sleep, and many other things. When you apply essential oils to the skin, they are absorbed into the bloodstream, and through inhalation, they go directly to the brain, which is why it is so important to use organic oils from reputable producers (I list a few of my favorites in the Resources section).

Essential oils play a big role in my beauty and wellness practices. They have helped me to rid my home of toxic cleaners, and they have enlivened my rituals with healing and fragrance. These are just a few of the ways I have incorporated them into my life.

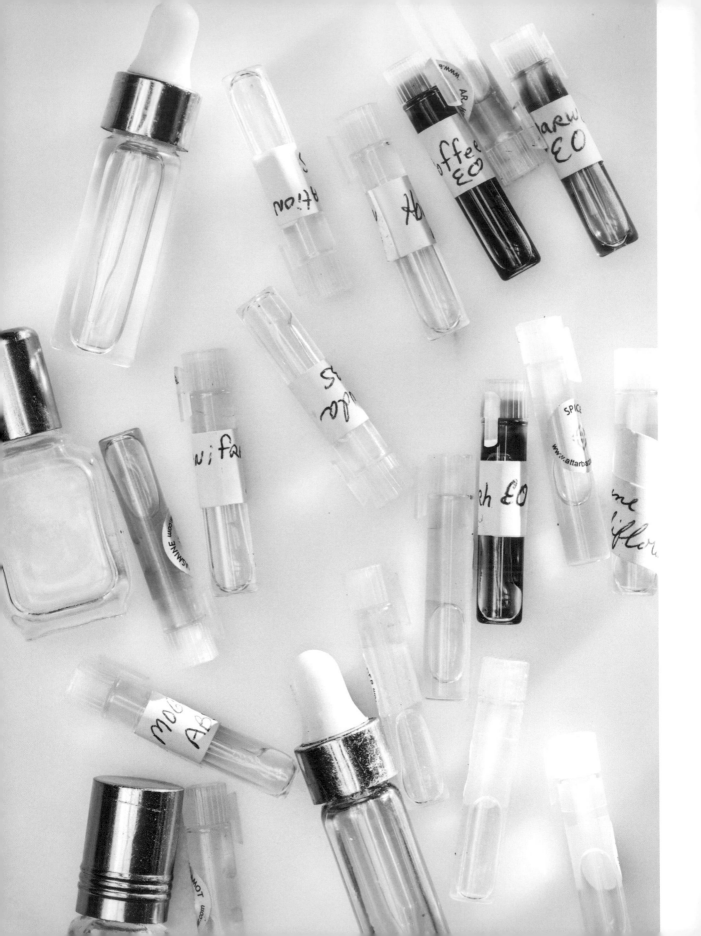

My Essential
Essential Oils

Essential oils are a remedy for everything from sleepless nights to sore muscles, headaches, cuts, and insect bites. Often, a simple inhalation does wonders, but you can also rub these oils directly on your body after diluting them with jojoba oil (check the label, as some are already diluted) so that they are absorbed into the skin.

They are lovely when applied to temples, the soles of the feet, pulse points, or pressure points. I use essential oils throughout my day: energizing and uplifting oils like peppermint and lemon in the morning; oils that help me focus and revive me on busy afternoons, like frankincense and sandalwood; and soothing, relaxing oils like lavender before going to bed or when I am traveling.

To inhale them, put a few drops on a cotton ball or a tissue, hold it to your face, and breath in deeply. Use them in an essential oil diffuser to scent a room or put a few drops in the linen closet.

Be sure to test your sensitivity to an essential oil by first applying a drop to the inside of your arm.

Following are the oils I like to have on hand.

Frankincense Oil

This ancient oil promotes an overall sense of well-being. It helps to relieve inflammation, boosts your immune system, aids in digestion after a heavy meal, and relieves and eases premenstrual symptoms and cramps. Its astringent properties help kill germs on the skin, and it has even been shown to fight some cancer cells.

Lavender Oil

Lavender oil is a go-to classic, but you can also choose a different flower oil, such as geranium, clary sage, rose, neroli, or jasmine. These oils will soothe your nerves and help you relax, and you can add drops to your skin and body oils, or anoint pulse points, to increase feelings of sensuality and attractiveness. Flower oils can help lift your mood and transition you back to your emotional and creative self after too many long hours at work. They also can be used to make closets and nurseries smell light and lovely.

Lemon Oil

Lemon oil is an instant mood booster. Massaging a few drops into the bottom of the feet can help wake you up when you're feeling sluggish. Lemon helps decongest the liver, balance blood sugar, and ease hunger. For people used to being in the spotlight, lemon helps them to find gratifying pathways and peace of mind without external validation, as it clears the auric fields and resets your olfactory senses. It is a great oil to take on vacation. I always have a bottle with me when I travel.

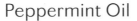

Peppermint Oil

Peppermint oil delivers an icy blast on a hot day.
Cooling and soothing, it helps alleviate muscle pain
and can calm an upset stomach or a throbbing
head. Breathing it in or massaging it into the chest
can help with respiratory issues from colds or
allergies. This is an oil that stimulates creativity.

Rosemary Oil

Rosemary oil relieves stress and anxiety while
boosting clarity and focus. It is a great aid when
studying for a test or preparing for a big event
that will require lots of concentration and planning.
It promotes physical stamina and emotional
strength. When massaged into the scalp, it
promotes hair growth and prevents dandruff, and
it also helps increase circulation, which makes it
a wonderful addition to massage and body oils.

Sandalwood Oil

If you can afford some high-quality sandalwood oil, it
is a sensual and luxurious addition to your essential-
oil regimen. It helps to relax breathing and serves
as an antidepressant. It increases vitality and is a
superior oil for meditation, as it helps you center
yourself and connect with the source of all being.

Tea Tree Oil

Tea tree oil is a wonderful alternative to antifungal
products. It is a powerful antiseptic that can be
used to treat acne, bacterial infections, insect
bites, dandruff, and fungal infections like candida,
nail fungus, and ringworm. *Note: While many
essential oils (like oregano or cinnamon) can be
taken internally, never ingest tea tree oil.*

Hydrosols

No matter what they might claim on the label, many modern moisturizers actually dry out your skin rather than nourish and nurture it. As we age, our skin stops producing as much oil, so we need to take extra care to replenish it, and spritzing throughout the day is a great way to help keep skin hydrated and supple. Hydrosols provide a centering burst of moisture and refreshment wherever you are and whenever you need it. I keep them in the car to bring a little peace when I'm stuck in traffic, and I take them when I travel by plane. I use them regularly to cool down on hot days, and also to clear space for meditation and rituals.

I encourage you to get creative, adapt, and play with the following recipes until you've made something that is uniquely perfect for you. Create whatever calls to you in that moment—maybe it's gold or amethyst— to soothe your skin and your soul. Adding crystals helps to enhance the desired vibrations and energy.

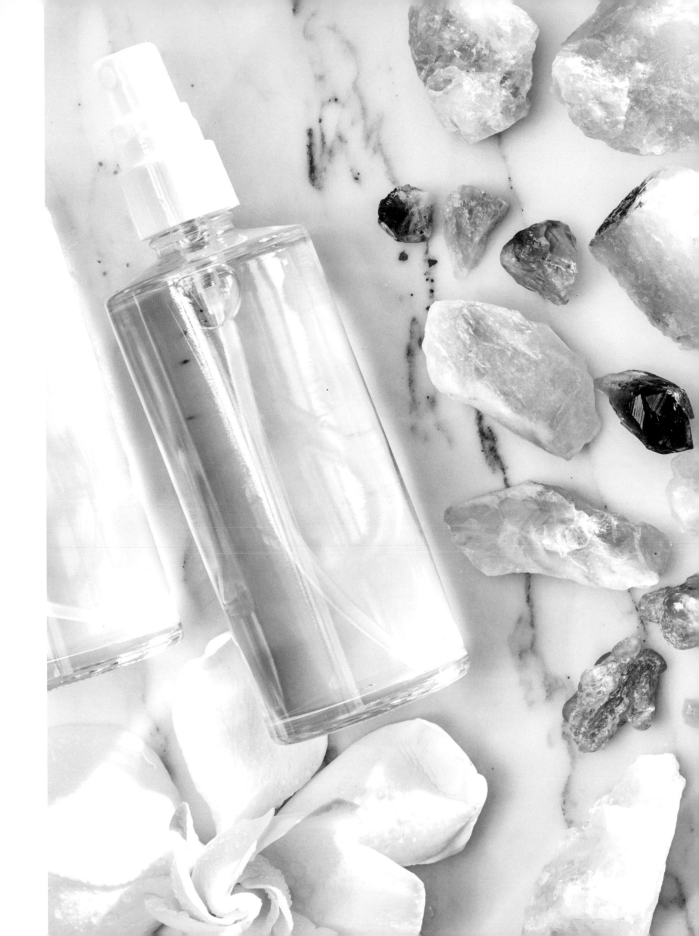

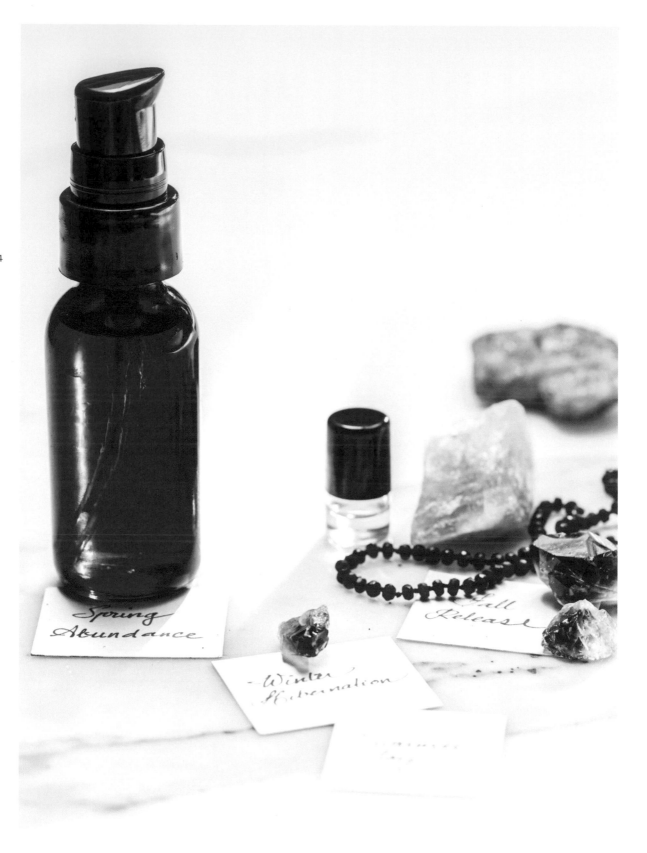

Seasonal Hydrosols

4 ounces purified water

1 drop of colloidal silver to act as a natural preservative (you can buy this at most health food stores)

Essential oils and crystals for the season of your choosing

Glass spray bottle

One way to balance your skin during changing weather is to use a specific hydrosol for the corresponding season.

Fill the spray bottle with the water and colloidal silver. Add the essential oils of your choosing and shake to mix. A good starting point is five drops of each oil, then you can add more of the individual oils until you've created a scent that is pleasing to you. Add the crystals and spritz as needed. You cannot overuse hydrosols. Stored out of the sun, they should last about a month.

SPRING ABUNDANCE

Essential Oils
Lily, neroli, rose,
sweet orange, sweet pea

Crystals
Amethyst for courage and
protection
Rose quartz for love and healing

SUMMER JOY

Essential Oils
Cucumber, gardenia, jasmine,
lavender, lemon, lemongrass,
mint, rose geranium, rosemary

Crystals
Moonstone for sleep and beauty
Watermelon tourmaline for
compassion and balance

FALL RELEASE

Essential Oils
Amber, oakmoss,
patchouli, sage, vanilla

Crystals
Black tourmaline for clearing negativity
Citrine for psychic awareness
Jade for longevity and prosperity

WINTER HIBERNATION

Essential Oils
Cedar, cinnamon, clove, cypress,
juniper, patchouli, pine, sandalwood

Crystals
Garnet for energy and to strengthen
your aura
Lemon quartz for clarity and abundance
Pearl for luck and money

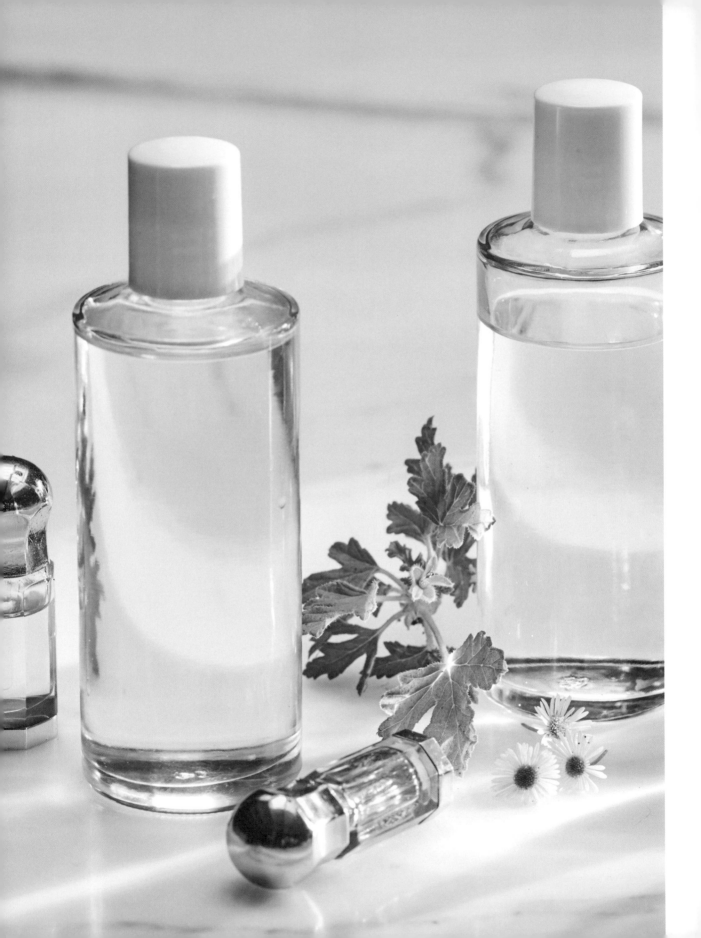

Toners

The microbiome of skin mirrors the
microbiome of soil. If you don't have
healthy soil, you won't have healthy food.
Just the same, if you don't have a healthy
microbiome on your face, you won't have
healthy skin. The microbiome is made
out of good bacteria, so you don't want
to strip it from your skin. Toners feed
your skin certain nutrient-rich elements,
which help to nourish the microbiome,
allowing it to flourish. This can ease
dry skin and help stop breakouts.

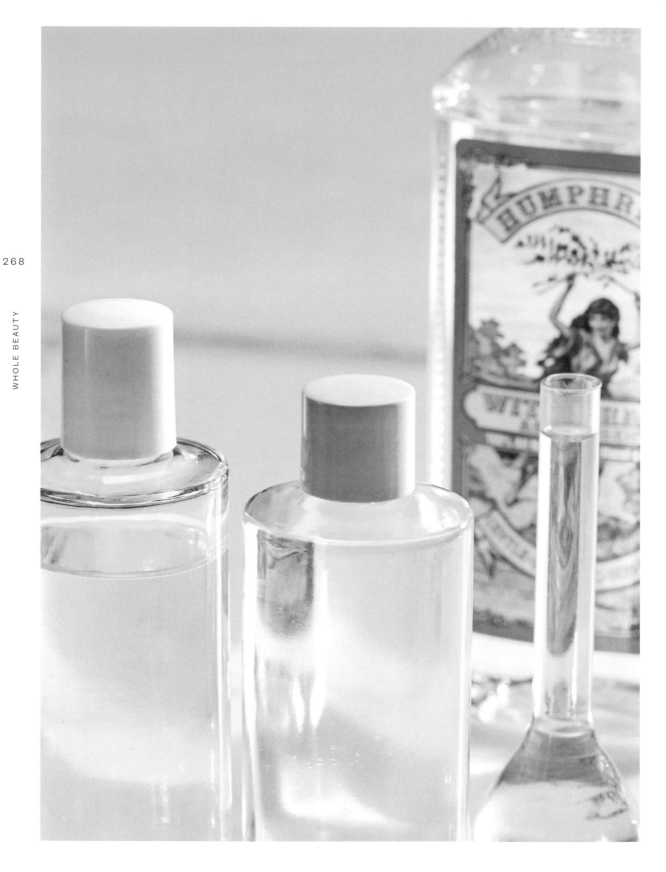

Toner Blends

6 ounces purified water

1 drop of colloidal silver to act as a
   natural preservative (you can buy
   this at most health food stores)

Ingredients for your skin type

Glass bottle with cap

For Normal / Combination Skin

1 tablespoon witch hazel

5 drops of lavender oil

3 drops of grapefruit oil

3 drops of Virginia cedarwood oil

For Acne-Prone / Oily Skin

1 tablespoon apple cider vinegar

5 drops of lavender oil

5 drops of tea tree oil

3 drops of grapefruit oil

2 drops of lemongrass oil

For Aging / Dry Skin

1 tablespoon aloe vera

10 drops of petitgrain

5 drops of frankincense

2 drops of geranium oil

2 drops of carrot seed oil (or 3 drops
   of Roman chamomile oil, if you
   don't like the carrot seed scent)

I apply toner after I cleanse and again after I put on an oil. Toners add minerals to the skin and set the groundwork for moisturizing, and they can also serve in a pinch when you can't do a full cleanse.

Put the water, colloidal silver, and ingredients that pertain to your skin type in the glass bottle. Tightly close the cap and shake to mix. Apply with a cotton pad. Store out of direct sunlight for up to 3 months.

Essential Oil Perfumes

In a time when almost every scent is recognizable, or easily accessible via the internet, why not create a signature scent that evokes where you are in the moment? Just like we can choose our outfits depending on our mood, we can do the same with hand-blended custom perfumes.

The beautiful thing about blending essential oil perfumes is that there is no right or wrong way to do it. You simply follow your nose until you have something that agrees with you. In this way, it is easy to create a signature scent, or you can combine different oils that you alternate depending on mood and occasions.

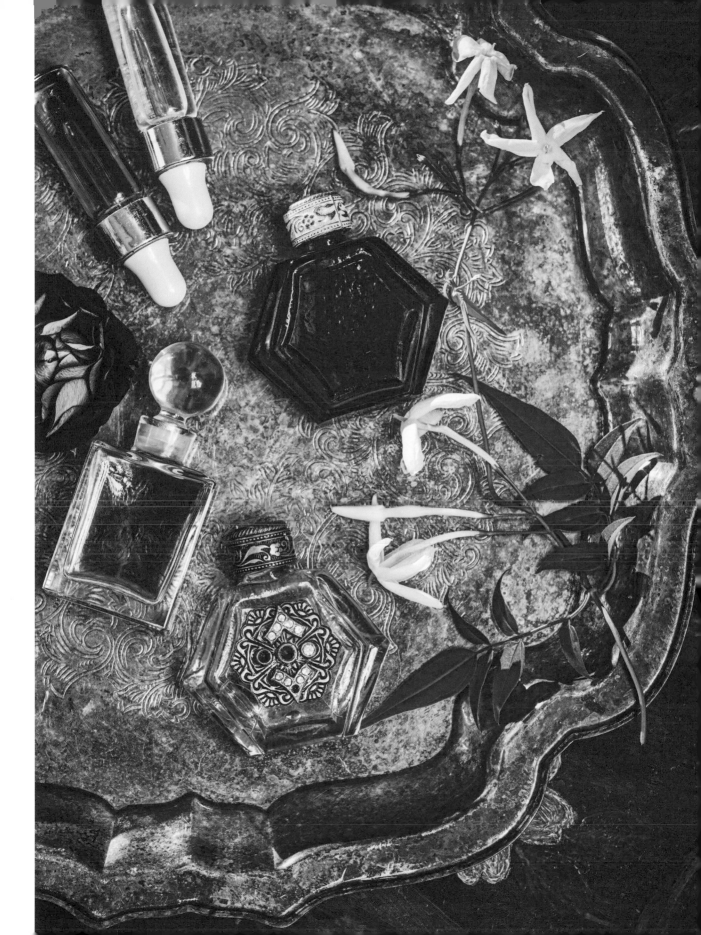

Goddess Perfumes

5 drops of each essential oil for the goddess of your choosing (or adjust to your preference)

1 tablespoon jojoba oil

Glass bottle with stopper or rollerball applicator (common sizes are 10 and 15 milliliters)

I love invoking the goddesses in my rituals, and I frequently set up their images and offerings on my altars. I created these perfume blends as a way to take the goddesses with me wherever I go. If I am standing in line, caught in traffic, or otherwise involved in a stressful situation, all I need to do is dab a little of one of these scents on my wrists to invoke Lalita's love or Artemis's courage. I blend them in front of my altar, on a Friday night to honor Venus, or during a waning moon, when the moon is preparing to renew. After the scent has been mixed, I will leave it on the altar for a few days to charge it with goddess energy.

Drop the essential oils of your choice into the glass bottle or rollerball applicator. Top with the jojoba oil. Tightly close the lid, and shake to mix. Charge it on your altar for a few days before applying. Store out of direct sunlight for up to 3 months.

Venus	Lakshmi	Artemis
Jasmine	Lily	Cedar
Rose	Rose	Frankincense
Ylang-ylang	Sandalwood	Juniper

Parvati	Freyja	Lalita
Cardamom	Musk	Amber
Vanilla	Patchouli	Musk
Ylang-ylang	Sandalwood	Vanilla

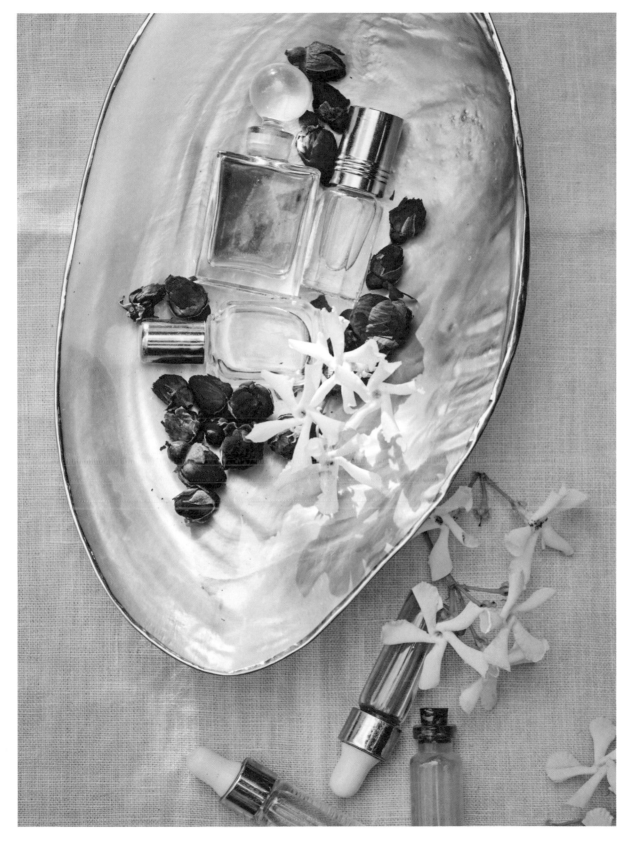

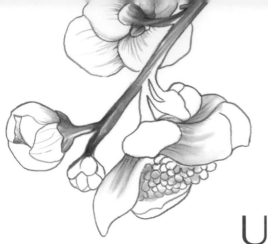

Using Essential Oils to Activate Your Chakras

Chakras can be activated through meditation and massage. Since the chakras are yearning to be opened and flowing, essential oils are a powerful tool to help this along. There are times when I feel ungrounded, so I reach for an earthy, wood-based essential oil. Just by placing a few drops on my feet, I feel a deeper connection to the earth. Or sometimes I place rose essential oil on my heart chakra, and my whole body softens. This is something you can experiment with; feel the subtle changes occurring with each use.

Our chakras will absorb everything, so using pure essential oils is a must.

CHAKRAS AND THEIR ESSENTIAL OILS

FIRST CHAKRA (ROOT)

Cedarwood · Myrrh · Patchouli

SECOND CHAKRA (SACRUM)

Bergamot · Clary Sage
Jasmine · Ylang-Ylang

THIRD CHAKRA (SOLAR PLEXUS)

Cinnamon · Geranium · Ginger · Juniper
Lemon · Rosemary · Sandalwood

FOURTH CHAKRA (HEART)

Cypress · Melissa ·Rose · Ylang-Ylang

FIFTH CHAKRA (THROAT)

Basil · Cypress · Chamomile
Palmarosa · Peppermint

SIXTH CHAKRA (THIRD EYE)

Bay · Cedarwood · Clary Sage
Frankincense · Helichrysum · Sandalwood

SEVENTH CHAKRA (CROWN)

Frankincense · Lavender
Myrrh · Sandalwood

Anointing Your Doshas

Anointing ourselves with essential oils is an empowering way to shift our energy and take control of our vision for what we want in our lives. It also can help to balance our doshas. To do this, I like to take a few drops of the appropriate oil on my finger, and start at the top of my head. I work down from the crown of my head, to my third eye, then my heart, right below my belly button, the pubic bone, and finally the soles of my feet. As I do so, I also imagine that I am activating my chakras and flooding them with pure, positive light.

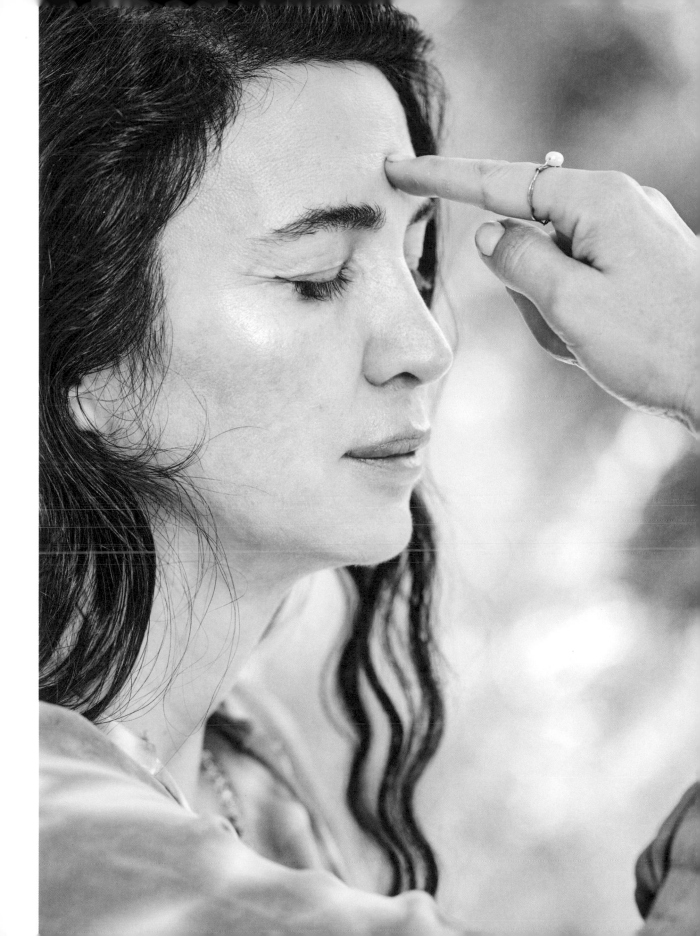

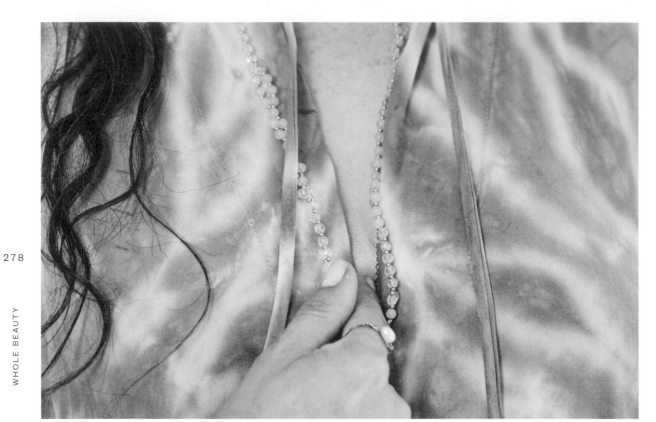

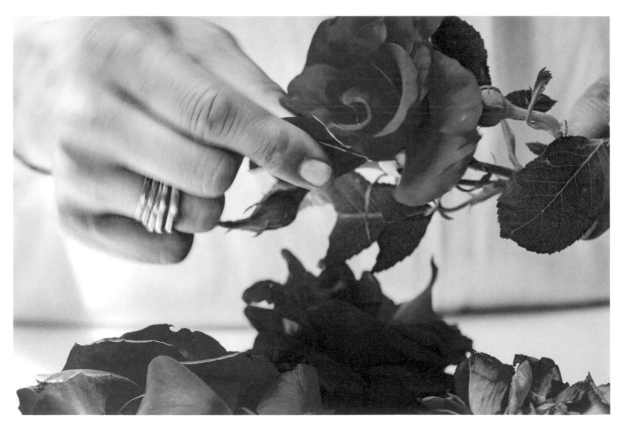

TO CALM VATA

Clary Sage · Geranium · Jasmine
Musk · Rose · Sandalwood

TO COOL PITTA

Gardenia · Jasmine
Melissa · Mint · Rose

TO STIMULATE KAPHA

Cedar · Cinnamon · Myrrh
Patchouli · Pine · Sage

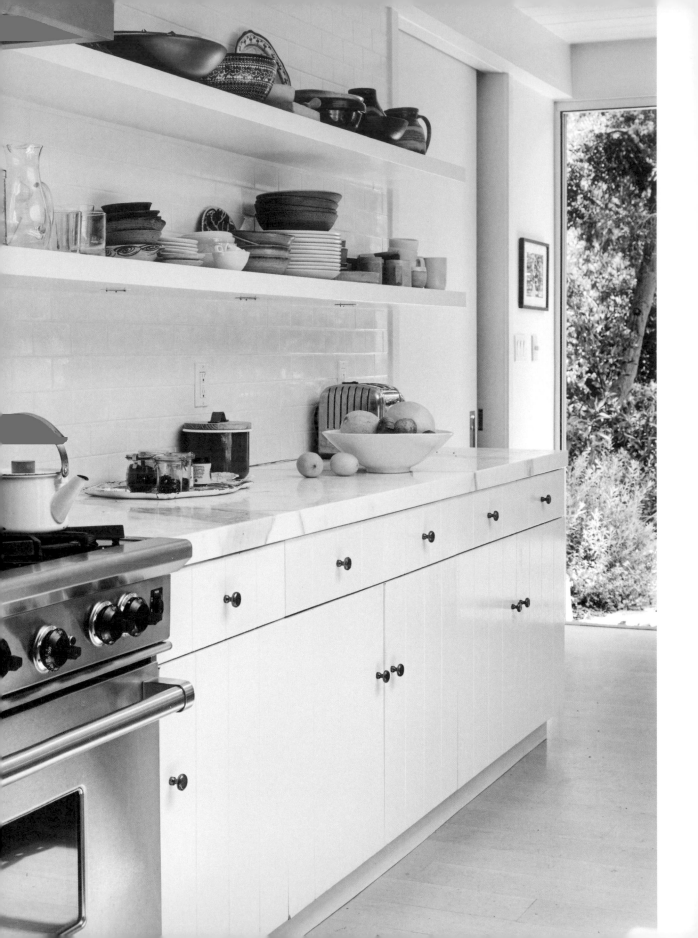

Essential Oils for Daily Use

Essential oils have been of great use to me in lessening my family's daily exposure to toxic chemicals in cleaning and personal care products. We absorb so much more than we are aware of, and to limit and ideally eliminate the hormone-disrupting chemicals is key to leading a life of health and vitality. These recipes smell clean and fresh and are also fun to make.

Deodorant

⅓ cup coconut oil, at room
    temperature
2 tablespoons organic baking soda
⅓ cup arrowroot powder (easy to
    find at health food stores)
8 drops of rose essential oil
8 drops of sandalwood essential oil

Mason jar

Around the age of twenty, I developed a lump beneath my armpit. There wasn't a ton of information about this at the time, but I began to do some research and became aware of the toxic implications of using traditional antiperspirants and deodorants made with aluminum. This was way back in the early nineties when there wasn't a Whole Foods on every corner, and the internet wasn't what it is today, so I began to hunt for more "natural" choices at mom-and-pop health food stores. All I could really find were the crystal kind—which didn't work—so I began to make my own, one of my first forays into DIY products. Shortly after I stopped using traditional antiperspirants, the lump disappeared. This recipe is for a deodorant, not an antiperspirant. As inconvenient as it may be at times, you want to sweat! Sweating is an important part of your body's detoxification process.

Place the coconut oil in a small bowl and add the baking soda and arrowroot powder. Mash together with a wooden spoon until the mixture has the consistency of deodorant (white and chalky, yet not too crumbly). Add the essential oils. Transfer to the mason jar and use your fingers to rub it under your arms until it is absorbed. Wait to dress until after it has dried, to avoid smearing it on your clothes. Stored out of direct sunlight, it will keep for 6 to 9 months.

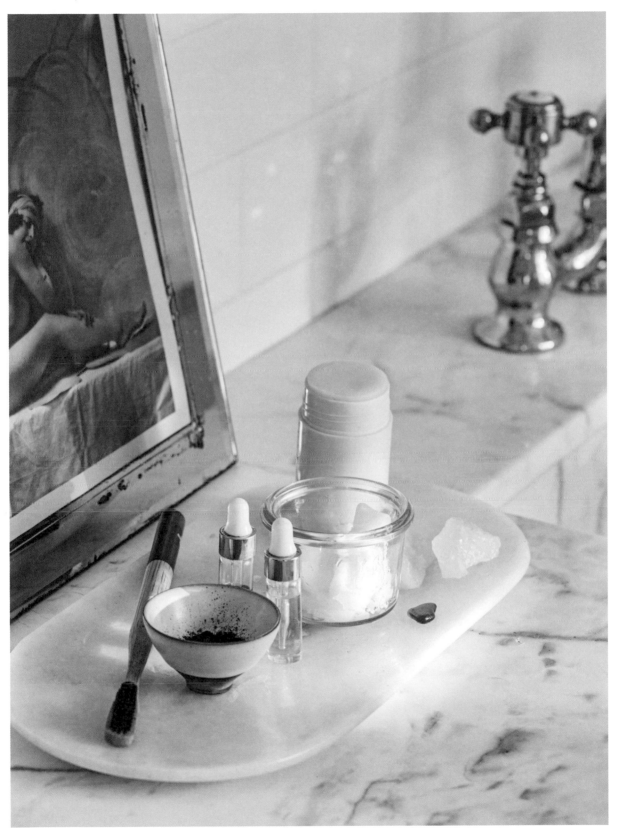

Toothpaste

3 tablespoons organic baking soda
3 tablespoons coconut oil
2 teaspoons glycerin
A few drops of stevia or 1 packet
   of xylitol (which also fights
   tooth decay)
20 drops of peppermint or
   cinnamon oil

Glass jar with lid

I am wary of overexposure to fluoride. You will be getting some naturally, as it is in the tap water, so having fluoride in your toothpaste is often redundant and could be harmful if not monitored. I like this tasty and refreshing DIY toothpaste, and my daughter Charlotte Rumi Rose loves making it with me. Coconut oil is known to be an antibacterial agent, and it helps fight tooth decay. To increase the whitening effect, you can add a drop of hydrogen peroxide to the paste.

Mix the baking soda, coconut oil, glycerin, and stevia or xylitol together (it helps if the coconut oil is a little warm; see page 202), then add the peppermint or cinnamon oil. Transfer to the glass jar. To use, dip your toothbrush into the jar. Stored out of direct sunlight, it will keep for 6 to 9 months.

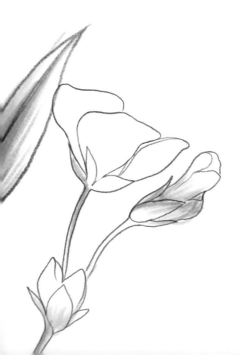

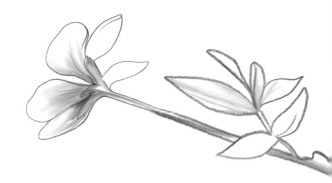

Insect Repellent

½ cup water
¼ cup witch hazel
45 drops of eucalyptus oil
30 drops of lemon oil
10 drops of peppermint oil

6-ounce glass spray bottle

A few summers ago, I was traveling to Kenya with a bunch of friends. Because of the many shots we were supposed to get and pills we were supposed to take just as a precaution, I almost decided not to go. Finally, I spoke to a friend who convinced me to reconsider. I used essential oils to repel mosquitoes, and got to experience an incredible trip, seeing wildlife and meeting beautiful people, without getting bitten once! Studies have since shown that blends of lemon and eucalyptus oils can repel mosquitoes as effectively as toxic DEET. As always, this is something you should discuss with your physician, as there are many serious bug-borne illnesses.

Combine the water and witch hazel with the eucalyptus, lemon, and peppermint oils in the spray bottle, and shake well before applying often. Stored out of direct sunlight, it will keep for 6 to 9 months.

Cleaning with Essential Oils

My aversion to toxic cleaning chemicals dates back to when I was five years old and my family was still living in Iran. Every evening, my father would come home from work and make himself a cocktail of vodka and orange juice. One day, when my parents were out, my three-year-old brother, Nader, decided to emulate his papa and make himself a drink. He found a bottle of bleach under the sink, poured some into a glass, mixed it with orange juice, and drank it.

My adopted older sister, Parvaneh, who was twelve at the time, acted quickly and instinctively when she saw the cabinet open and Nader sitting there with the bleach. She saved his life. Parvaneh (which

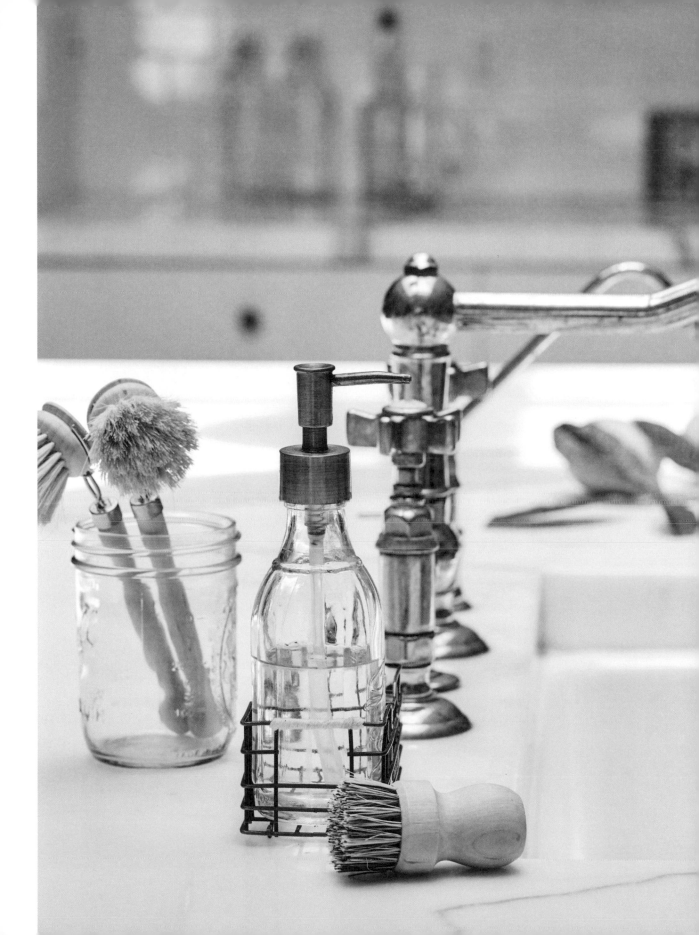

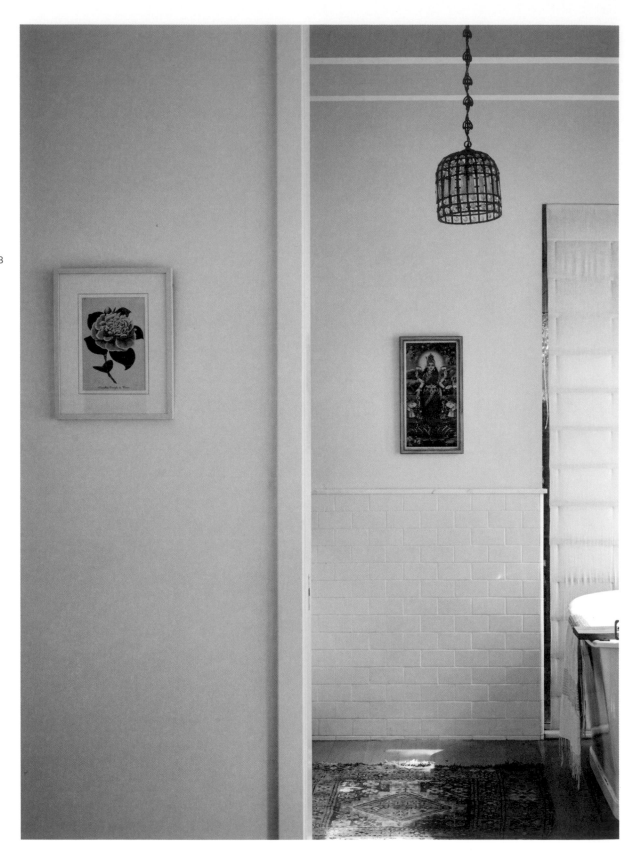

means "butterfly" in Farsi) had been raised in a nearby village, but her parents had decided to sell her off as a bride. My parents, shocked at this barbarity, "bought" her for a few dollars and brought her to live as their daughter.

Parvaneh had seen shepherds feed their sheep yogurt when the sheep had eaten something that made them sick. Immediately after Nader drank the bleach, Parvaneh made him start eating yogurt and wouldn't let him stop. It coated his intestines and protected them from the corrosive bleach until my parents were able to get him to the nearest hospital, an hour away, to have his stomach pumped. Without Parvaneh's quick thinking, my brother surely would have died, and I can't help but feel that it was karma coming back to my parents for stepping up to adopt a village girl. Morals of the story: Don't keep chemicals under the sink, keep pure yogurt in the fridge, and you never know how one kind gesture can shape your whole life in the future.

Note that in spite of their name, essential oils are rarely oily, so don't worry about using them in the following preparations. They won't leave a greasy film behind.

Dishwashing Liquid

2 cups water
¼ cup soap flakes
¼ cup castile soap (I like Dr. Bronner's)
1 teaspoon glycerin
2 teaspoons washing soda (easy to find at hardware stores or superstores)
Essential oils of your choosing (see below)

Glass bottle with spout

For a Citrus Version
15 drops of grapefruit oil
15 drops of lemon oil

For an Evergreen Version
15 drops of cedar oil
15 drops of juniper oil

For a Floral Version
15 drops of geranium oil
15 drops of lavender oil

Bring the water to a low boil in a pot, then add the soap flakes and stir until they're dissolved. Remove from the heat to let cool, add the castile soap, glycerin, washing soda, and the essential oils of your choosing, and pour into the glass bottle. Shake well before each use. Stored out of direct sunlight, it will keep for up to 6 months.

Surface & Floor Cleaner

½ cup white vinegar
½ gallon water
2 tablespoons organic baking soda
Essential oils of your choosing
(see below)

Glass spray bottle (you can also use
plastic, but I prefer glass to avoid
exposure to phthalates and BPA)
or metal bucket

For a Citrus Version
10 drops of grapefruit oil
10 drops of lemon oil

For an Evergreen Version
10 drops of cedar oil
10 drops of juniper oil

For a Floral Version
10 drops of geranium oil
10 drops of lavender oil

Mix the vinegar, water, and baking soda in the spray bottle or bucket, and add the essential oils of your choosing. To use, shake or stir well, then apply and wipe or mop clean. Stored out of direct sunlight, it will keep for up to 6 months.

Bleach Alternative

10 cups water
¼ cup lemon juice
1 cup hydrogen peroxide
10 drops of lemon oil

Water jug

Mix the water, lemon juice, hydrogen peroxide, and lemon oil in the water jug, and use 1 cup for each load of whites. Stored out of direct sunlight, it will keep for up to 6 months.

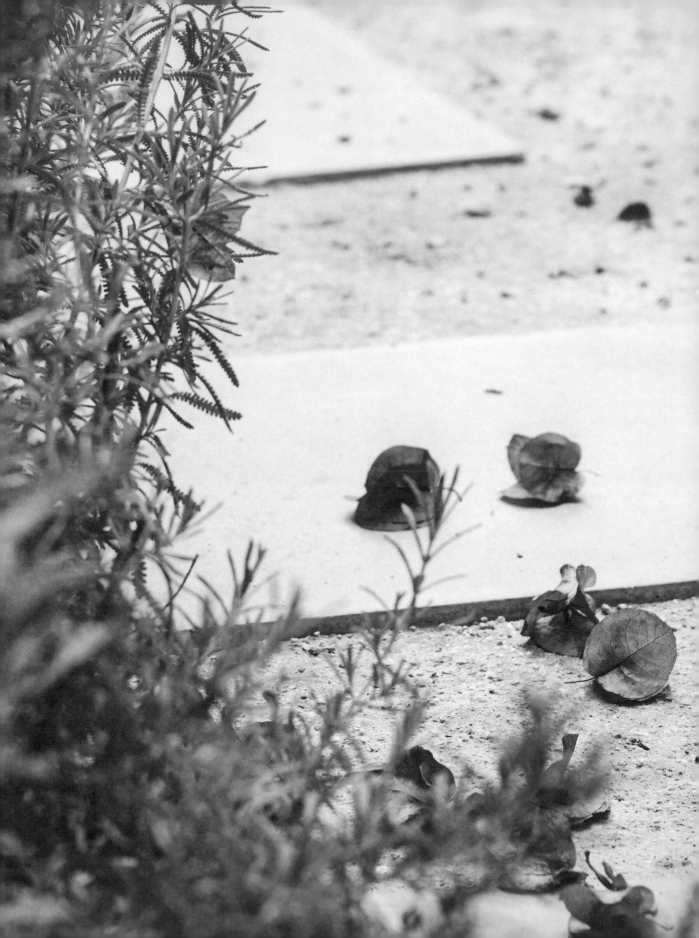

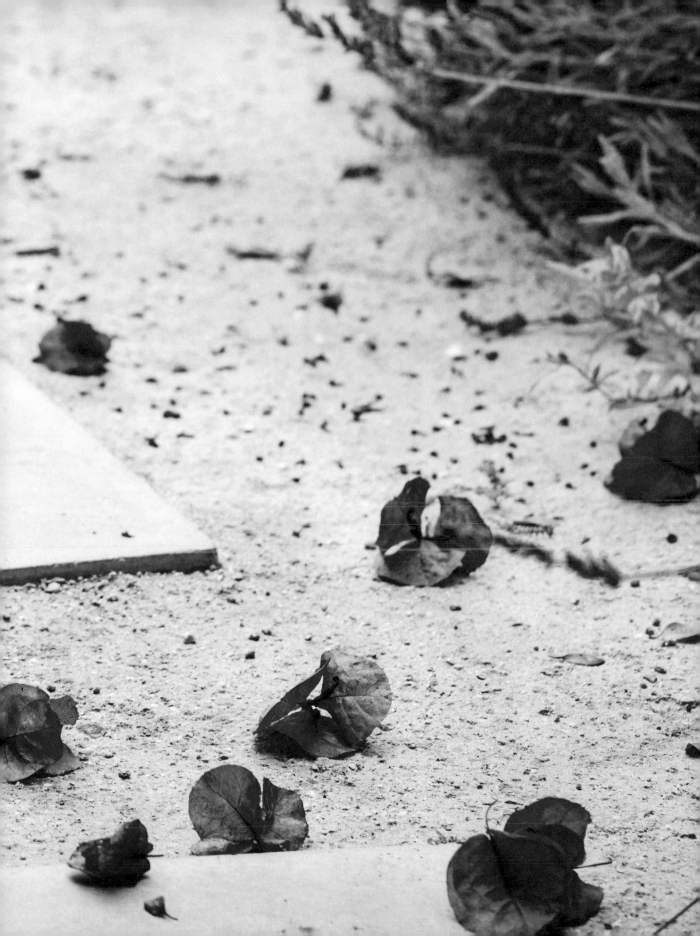

AFTERWORD

Recently, I found myself driving across the barren land of New Mexico from Ojo Caliente to Taos, and I was completely awestruck by the sunset. The sky was an incredible mix of blues, oranges, violets, and yellows, and as the beaming orb of the sun began to dip below the horizon, the sage bushes took on an ethereal glow.

As I drove, I became so overwhelmed with the beauty of the sky and land that I had to pull over to the side of the road and weep with gratitude for all that I was witnessing. In that moment, I recognized how much I have been transformed by the way I have been living. Rituals, practices, and being more present in nature have made me see the world with new eyes. I'm not sure if I would have really felt the bliss of that sunset in my former life. I realized that to see and feel the magic around us is truly what it means to be content and fulfilled.

Thank you so much for trusting me to take you on this journey, as this has been a culmination of so many of the passions and healings that have been important to me over the past few years. I hope that I can bring some awareness to this world and illuminate it for you, and that this book will serve as a bridge to a new place of spirituality and beauty—and a return to our true state of being, which is alive, healthy, blissful, vibrant, and whole. Writing *Whole Beauty* has truly been a labor of love, and I am so deeply grateful for all the challenges and all the blessings that have led me down this path.

I continue to learn something new every day as my path spirals and unwinds, and I am constantly reminded to stay curious and never lose the wonder I had as a child. We must be grateful for the little things in our lives that are above, below, and beside us. We must always see the beauty. I hope this book brings you some pleasure, light, and peace, and that your journey will transform your life in the same way mine did for me.

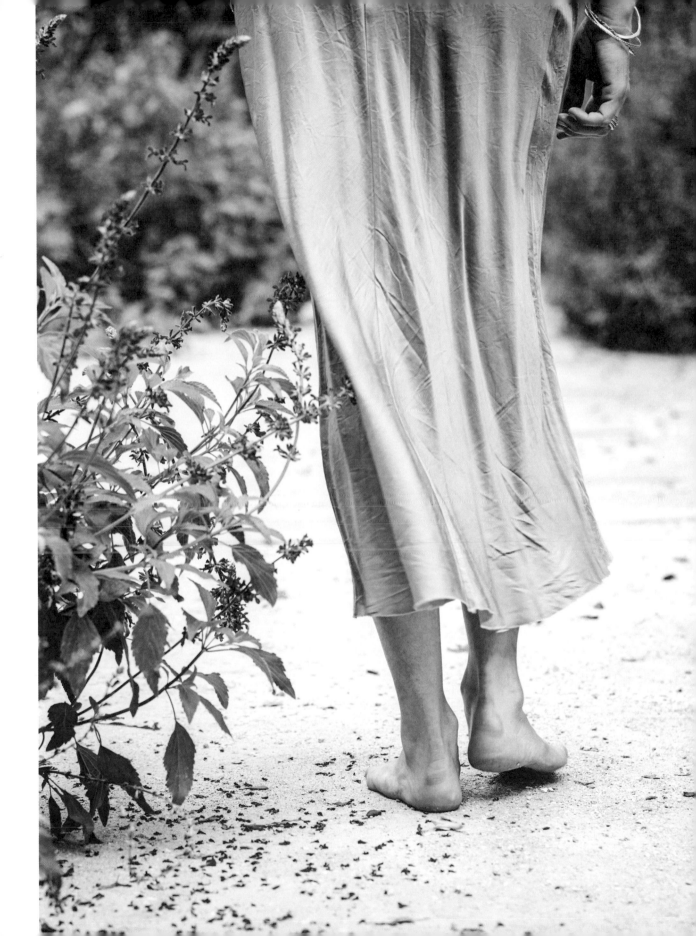

FURTHER READING

IN ADDITION TO IN MY BLOG, *THE LOCAL ROSE*, MY
WRITING HAS APPEARED ON THE FOLLOWING WEBSITES.

TheChalkboardMag.com
Goop.com
MindBodyGreen.com

THESE ARE THE BOOKS THAT I PULL OFF
THE SHELF AGAIN AND AGAIN.

*Awakening Shakti: The Transformative Power of
the Goddesses of Yoga*, by Sally Kempton

*Ayurvedic Beauty Care: Ageless Techniques to
Invoke Natural Beauty*, by Melanie Sachs

*The Complete Book of Essential Oils and
Aromatherapy,* by Valerie Ann Worwood

*The Goddess Pages: A Divine Guide to Finding Love
and Happiness*, by Laurie Sue Brockway

*Invincible Living: The Power of Yoga, the Energy of Breath,
and Other Tools for a Radiant Life*, by Guru Jagat

Love Is in the Earth: A Kaleidoscope of Crystals, by Melody

Magical Herbalism: The Secret Craft of the Wise,
by Scott Cunningham

Natural Organic Hair and Skin Care, by Aubrey Hampton

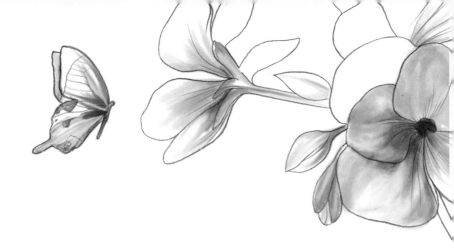

RESOURCES

LEARN MORE ABOUT HOLISTIC LIVING AND MY PRODUCTS ON THELOCALROSE.COM. IN ADDITION, THESE ARE THE WEBSITES I FREQUENTLY VISIT TO SHOP FOR INGREDIENTS AND SEEK NEW INSIGHTS AND INFORMATION.

Ayurveda
BanyanBotanicals.com
Chopra.com
SuryaSpa.com

To find an Ayurvedic practitioner in your area:
AyurvedaNAMA.org

Crystals
CrystalsMtShasta.com

Essential Oils
EdensGarden.com
LivingLibations.com

Ghee
AncientOrganics.com
FourthAndHeart.com

Herbs
BanyanBotanicals.com
DualSpices.com
MountainRoseHerbs.com
SusunWeed.com

Incense
BodhaModernWellness.com
EarthAndElement.com

Kundalini
GoldenBridgeYoga.com
RAMAYogaInstitute.com
3HO.org

Mantras
SpiritVoyage.com
WhiteSun.com

Nontoxic Makeup
IliaBeauty.com
KosasCosmetics.com
RMSBeauty.com
VapourBeauty.com

Spices and Ingredients
BanyanBotanicals.com
DualSpices.com

Tea Ceremony
GlobalTeaHut.org
LivingTea.net

Tonics
DragonHerbs.com
GoldenLotusHerbs.com
SunPotion.com

Yoni Eggs
KimAnami.com
DawnCartwright.com
LaylaMartin.com
SaidaDesilets.com

ACKNOWLEDGMENTS

I feel utterly grateful to those who made this journey from a dream in my mind to a tangible book manifest. To the beautiful Lia Ronnen at Artisan, who is keeping our culture afloat with books of beauty. And to her incredible team that made *Whole Beauty* become whole: Shoshana Gutmajer, who has been incredibly insightful, patient, and supportive; Charlotte Heal, who captured the essence of the book through her imaginative design; Sibylle Kazeroid; Michelle Ishay-Cohen; Renata Di Biase; Nancy Murray; Hanh Le; Elise Ramsbottom; and Allison McGeehon.

To my book agents, Meg Thompson and Cindy Uh. Meg, I am so grateful to you for believing in my story and vision from the beginning, without ever once wavering. To Kate Williams for structuring my wanderings. To Ngoc Minh Ngo, whose eye and steady hand captures the natural world in all its delicate, fleeting beauty.

Thank you to my parents, who loved me into being. The adventure between a charismatic Persian man and a beauty queen from Millbrae, California, began long ago. Their love crossed oceans and boundaries at a time when that was unheard of, and from that union came my dear younger brother, Nader, and me.

To my daughters, who make me strive to become a better human being. Colette for teaching me gentility and the lightness of being. Charlotte for teaching me to dig in the soil, and to dig even deeper in my soul.

To the women who are always there for me and teach me all the ways of being in the world: Lilakoi Moon for showing me what regality really means; Rosetta Getty for showing me gentle elegance; Jena King for showing me generosity of heart.

To the community of like-minded sisters who are bringing great changes to this planet: Nitsa Citrine (pictured on page 218), Tien Wu (Baelyn Elspeth; pictured on page 106), Mystic Mama (Mijanou Montealegre), Daughter of the Sun (Amy Woodruff), Nadine Artemis, Yvonne Gallegos, Mia Maestro, Bunni Nishimura,

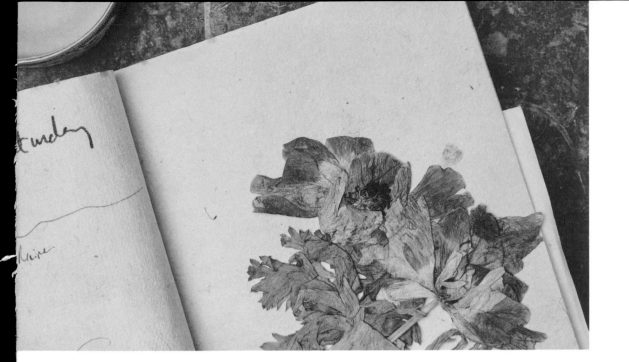

GianPrem (Jessica Suda), Jaclyn Hodes, Jessika Le Corre, GuruJas Khalsa, Shalom Harlow, Lacy Phillips, Wendy Plumb, Carolyn Murphy, Darby Hanon, Sam Barnouin, Jackie Rose, Jenni Kayne, Nicole Simone, Garance Doré, Athena Calderone, Amanda Chantal Bacon, and Jessica Karr—and to Eve Ensler for paving the way.

Thank you to the sacred masculine that is among us in its container of strength and stability. Thank you for your quiet courage and support of the divine feminine.

To my community of teachers, healers and friends: Dr. Soram Khalsa, who was on the holistic path before many of us were brave enough to venture there. Sanford Ponderson, who has given me a vast education with his healing sessions. Grace Vieira, who taught me the mantra "I say yes to life, and life says yes to me." Harijiwan Khalsa, who shares superpowers with his students. Guru Jagat, who teaches us how to be blissful, fierce, and wise. Harbhajian Singh Khalsa, who brought us powerful teachings to change our lives.

Wu De, who offers us the gifts of tea and meditation with his authentic presence. Nathan Bogle for being there, and being "on the bench." Euphemia Mendes for being family. Dylan McDermott for being father to our daugthers. Daneen Flesher, Katie Rayle, and Andre Melznick for putting me back together when my limbs gave up. The organic farmers in my area who have fed my family and me for decades. The SGI community for teaching me that we can indeed turn poison into medicine.

Thank you to those who have been reading The Local Rose for years since its inception. Thank you to all who support my beauty line, and my teams at David Pirrotta and Elco Fulfillment, who work tirelessly behind the scenes to bring nontoxic beauty to the world. Also thank you to Carrie Pollare, Matt Fishburn, and Brian Scott.

Thank you lastly to Gaia, this beautiful earth, and to the sacred nourishing waters, the celestial realms, the goddesses, the trees, our plant allies, my guides, and the animals.

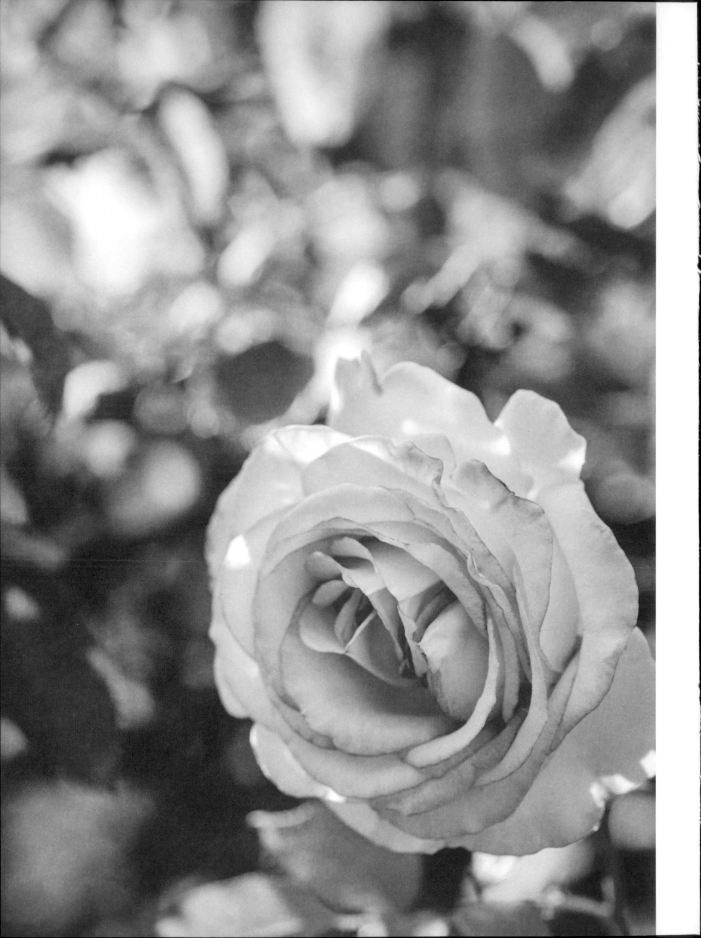

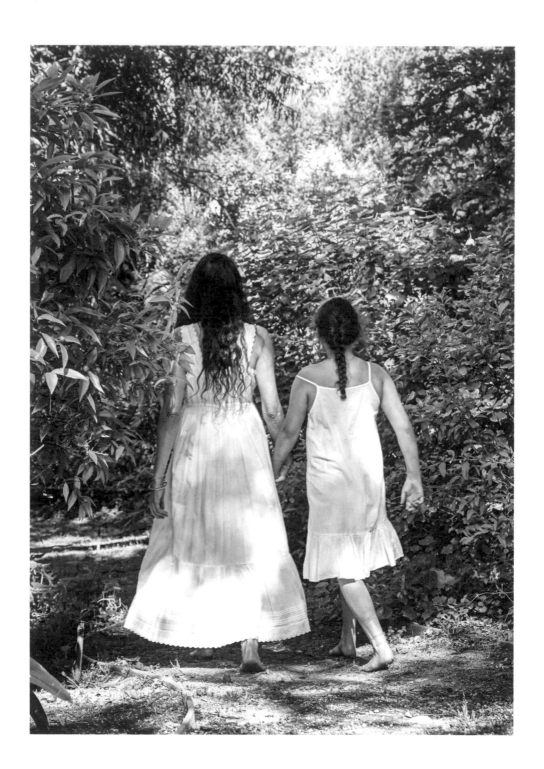